The Theory and Practice of

TAIJI QIGONG

Fourth Edition

Chris Jarmey

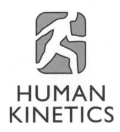

HUMAN
KINETICS

This fourth edition published in 2024 by
Lotus Publishing
Apple Tree Cottage, Inlands Road, Nutbourne, Chichester, PO18 8RJ, and
Human Kinetics
1607 N. Market Street, Champaign, Illinois 61820

United States and International
Website: **US.HumanKinetics.com**
Email: info@hkusa.com
Phone: 1-800-747-4457

Canada
Website: **Canada.HumanKinetics.com**
Email: info@hkcanada.com

Disclaimer
This publication is written and published to provide accurate and authoritative information relevant to the subject matter presented. It is published and sold with the understanding that the author and publisher are not engaged in rendering legal, medical, or other professional services by reason of their authorship or publication of this work. If medical or other expert assistance is required, the services of a competent professional person should be sought.

Drawings Bryan Nuttall
Text Design Medlar Publishing Solutions Pvt Ltd., India
Cover Design Chris Fulcher
Printed and Bound Kultur Sanat Printing House, Turkey

British Library Cataloguing-in-Publication Data
A CIP record for this book is available from the British Library

Library of Congress Cataloging-in-Publication Data
Names: Jarmey, Chris, author.
Title: The theory and practice of taiji qigong / Chris Jarmey.
Description: Fourth edition. | Champaign, Illinois : Human Kinetics, 2024.
Identifiers: LCCN 2023030193 (print) | LCCN 2023030194 (ebook) |
    ISBN 9781718231009 (paperback) | ISBN 9781718231016 (epub) |
    ISBN 9781718231023 (pdf)
Subjects: LCSH: Tai chi. | Qi gong.
Classification: LCC GV504 .J37 2023 (print) | LCC GV504 (ebook) |
    DDC 613.7/148--dc23/eng/20230808
LC record available at https://lccn.loc.gov/2023030193
LC ebook record available at https://lccn.loc.gov/2023030194

ISBN: 978-1-7182-3100-9
10 9 8 7 6 5 4 3 2 1

Contents

About the Author

C hris Jarmey, who tragically died prematurely in 2008, first became interested in Oriental philosophies at the age of 9, being particularly drawn to Buddhist and Daoist practices. This led him at the age of 14 into the exploration and practice of both Indian yoga and a Chinese martial art known as Kenpo.

His interest in practices that enhance or restore health was catalyzed at the age of 11, when he suffered a serious fall from a cliff face, damaging his pelvis and thoracic spine. This caused serious pain and mobility problems by the time he was 18, at which time he applied his budding understanding and experience of yoga and Qigong to successfully correct the problem. From then onwards his interest in the healing arts developed and he embarked upon a search for those who could teach him more about oriental healing methods.

Throughout the next 30 plus years, Chris Jarmey spent his time researching and practicing bodywork-based healing methods alongside the extensive practice of Buddhist and Daoist Qigong, yoga, and meditation methods. He was taught by several teachers, but considered himself particularly fortunate to have studied under Geshe Damcho Yonten (Tibetan Buddhism and meditation); Mother Sayama (Theravadan Vipassana meditation); Masahiro Oki (Dao-Yinn, Qigong, Shiatsu and Zen meditation); BKS Iyengar (Hatha Yoga); Okudo Roshi (Zen meditation); Dr Norman Allen (Ashtanga Yoga) and Pauline Sasaki (Shiatsu). Also of great value was information and insight gained at courses given by Dr. Shen Hongxun (Buqi and Qigong); Dr. Yang Jwing-Ming (Qigong); Master Mantak Chia (Qigong); and Dr. John Peacock (Kum Nye: Tibetan Yoga / Qigong).

In 1975, Chris began his study of Western approaches to healing and rehabilitation, as a means to contrast and supplement his experience of Eastern methods. He qualified as a state registered physiotherapist in 1978, with a special interest in therapeutic exercise systems. Shortly afterwards he embarked upon extensive study and research into osteopathic methodology. This was followed up with a training given by Carlo Depaoli in Western herbal medicine based on Traditional Chinese Medicine principles.

Concurrent with the above studies, from 1978 to 1981 he researched and evaluated the healing effects of yoga, shiatsu, and Qigong within NHS hospitals and medical rehabilitation centers, with good results.

Between 1981 and 1985 Chris lived and studied in a number of yoga centers and ashrams in India, the UK, and the USA, to broaden and deepen his experience of Indian Hatha Yoga and related arts, such as the ancient and comprehensive Indian medicine system known as Yoga Chikitsa. Then, in late 1985 he founded The European Shiatsu School to offer a comprehensive practitioner training course in this effective form of bodywork.

Acknowledgements

Firstly, I would like to express my gratitude to all the teachers and practitioners of Qigong, meditation, and the healing arts who have positively influenced my understanding and practice of those disciplines. I would like to thank Bryan Nuttall for the drawings; Jane Pollard for her insights into Yin-Yang theory and for allowing the use of some of her collated material on that subject; Liz Welch, Isabelle Mazille and Bryan Nuttall for modeling the Qigong exercises; also Liz Welch, and Bryan Nuttall for offering their constructive views on some of the nuances and contradictions within Qigong theory.

In addition I wish to thank George Dellar; Debbie Jarmey; Susan Millington Ph.D., Bryan Nuttall; Jane Pollard; Andrea Smith Ph.D., and Liz Welch for proof reading the manuscript.

How to Use This Book

This book acts as an in-depth instruction manual for the practice of the 18 Stances of Taiji Qigong (Taiji Qigong Shibashi), which is widely practiced throughout the Far East and increasingly throughout the Western world. Many of the exercises are loosely based on the movements and stances of Taiji Quan. However, it is not to be confused with Qigong exercises for Taiji Quan, although it could be used as such.

Methods of Qigong are many, and the variations within these methods are endless. Even within Taiji Qigong Shibashi there are at least six different "styles" that I have come across; which means there must be even more. Generally though, this method of Qigong and its variations are practiced as a very simple, easy to learn system that is ideal for beginners. However, many people also use it as a serious core practice, or as an adjunct to yet deeper methods.

This book is written with all levels and depths of practice in mind. It is constructed so that you can take from it the necessary information and techniques to suit your goals. If you want to use it as a basic Qigong health and well-being maintenance program, you can largely ignore Part 1 and go straight to Parts 2 and 3.

If you want to practice with a view to really experiencing your internal energy, read Part 1, but understand that some theories and practices described belong to deeper levels of Qigong and are mentioned purely to put this level of training into context and give a broad overview. If you are an experienced practitioner of the deeper internal methods of Qigong, Part 1 may serve to clarify certain concepts for you, and enable you to apply some of those internal methods to Taiji Qigong. The so-called "levels" or depths of practice are not meant to imply a greater or lesser quality of practice. They simply relate to one's goals. There are many benefits to be gained from practicing what appears to be a more external, simple system, and many pitfalls to practicing more complex or deeper techniques. This is because the consequences of practicing incorrectly are greater; which can easily happen without a good teacher monitoring your work.

So, when you get to Part 3, follow the general instructions, but when you get to mental focus, choose either basic, intermediate, or advanced focus according to your experience and aspirations. Basic focus represents the focus used by the vast majority of people who do these exercises. Intermediate focus is for those who want to explore the power of their visualization skills within the exercises. Advanced focus is for experienced Qigong practitioners who are at least competent with reverse abdominal breathing (*see* page 62), and who wish to experience their internal movement and distribution of Qi at a deeper level.

Although the 18 stances are presented and commonly practiced as a unified set or "form", any of the exercises can be done in isolation or grouped together in smaller sets of your choice. However, if you find that you are consistently abandoning a particular exercise, just be aware that it is human nature to avoid the things that may ultimately allow us to grow.

It may be that you flick through this book and wonder why it has to be so detailed and "wordy". Is it not better to lean towards minimalism with regard to theory and instruction when dealing with what is essentially an experiential art? Shouldn't the individual be left to discover the effects, benefits, and effective mental focus through their own diligent practice? In a way, yes; and you can still take that approach with this book by simply following the instructions on how to move during each exercise.

However, the detail given beyond that is designed to offer ideas and indications that will speed up your progress. Believe nothing until you have tried it; and once you have experienced the subtleties for yourself, feel free to modify it, so long as you stay within the principles of Qi and Yin-Yang, which themselves have been tested and refined over many thousands of years.

PART I

The Theory of
Qi and Qigong

Taiji Qigong is an easy-to-learn system of energy enhancing exercises that co-ordinates movement with breathing and inner concentration. If practiced regularly, it will give you more energy, improve health, and help prevent illness. The primary aim of practicing this Qigong is to gently build and regulate your vitality by enhancing your Qi.

This method is uncomplicated to learn so most people should be able to master the basic movements within a week or so of regular practice. Mastering the subtleties and nuances will take considerably longer, but are well within the grasp of the keen student living the modern pace of life.

Within the full spectrum of possible Qigong methods, Taiji Qigong Shibashi has often been described as a relatively superficial system. However, if the nuances and subtleties are understood and practiced correctly, this Qigong becomes an ideal intermediate method of Qigong for anyone willing to do it on a daily basis. It is not one of the deeper internal methods fraught with life threatening consequences if mistakes are made; neither is it just a physical exercise. I would describe it as a realistic method for those who must practice largely unsupervised, but who wish to make real progress in the enhancement of their vitality.

If you work within any of the healing professions you will find Taiji Qigong an excellent adjunct to your work, because you will be giving out a lot of your energy in the form of compassion, concentration, and intent to heal when dealing with the illnesses of your patients. Taiji Qigong is particularly effective in helping to replenish that "giving" energy. It will also build energy (Qi) in your hands, which is particularly useful if you are a bodywork therapist. Taiji Qigong is also an excellent self-healing system to recommend to those you are trying to help.

■ What Is Qi?

Qi as a Universal Concept

Qi as a broad concept is the sub-strata of the entire universe. It includes everything in the universe from the most material to the immaterial. Therefore, within its broadest possible definition, we can consider a rock as Qi and we can consider an individual thought to be Qi. However, in practice, Qi is generally thought of as the invisible factors that bind matter together and activate all things, including those that are tangible but invisible to our senses. Visible and palpable things such as rocks are collectively known as Xing, whereas amorphous invisible phenomena such as wind, smell, heat, movement, or even happiness all fall under the general heading of Qi. Therefore to physically exist requires Qi, to move and feel requires Qi, and to think requires Qi.

You could say that Xing are all those things you can perceive and count, whereas Qi is all that which you cannot see or count. Another angle on this way of perceiving the universe is to consider that initially, things in the Xing category seem permanent, but the fact that all things are impermanent shows that they are constantly subject to change, however imperceptible that change may seem. The agents of change are those invisible factors called Qi.

Traditional Chinese philosophy considers the universe to be driven by three manifestations of Qi: Heaven Qi (Tian Qi), Earth Qi (Di Qi), and Human Qi (Ren Qi). Heaven Qi is the largest and most powerful of these forces, because it contains Earth Qi within it (the Earth itself being a planet within the heavens). Earth Qi is regarded as the aggregate of the earth's magnetic field and underground heat, which is believed to produce a matrix of energy lines and zones across and through the planet. Earthquakes and volcanic activity are thus seen as the Earth Qi re-balancing itself.

From our point of view, i.e., as beings standing upon this planet, Heaven Qi is considered to be the combined forces from above that exert influence upon the earth. This includes energy, gravity, and light from the sun, moon, and stars; forces which in turn govern climate. Climate, like everything else, is subject to fluctuation. So extremes of weather, including tornadoes, torrential rain, and so on are seen as Heaven Qi trying to restore balance.

The interaction of Heaven Qi with Earth Qi can be observed in other examples, such as too much heat from the sun and too little rain causing crops to fail in a drought. Thus it can be said that Earth Qi absorbs Heaven Qi and is influenced by it. Human Qi (and also Animal Qi) is seen as a melding of the forces of Heaven Qi and Earth Qi (Figure 1). Human Qi is

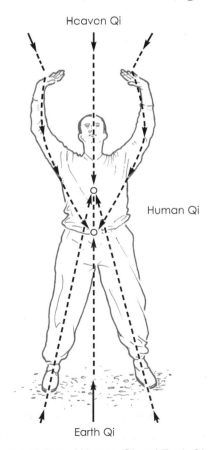

Figure 1: *Human Qi as a melding of Heaven Qi and Earth Qi.*

a type of energy field that draws Heaven Qi downward from above and Earth Qi upward from below. The balance of our Human Qi is therefore strongly influenced by the natural cycles of Heaven Qi and Earth Qi.

Harmonizing ourselves with the forces and cycles of Heaven and Earth is the core philosophy of Daoism from which Qigong developed. Daoists have observed that nature is a process of perpetual decay and renewal, and if you carefully observe nature, you can gain insight into the way nature cyclically re-balances its Qi. Daoist philosophy, within which the bulk of oriental medicine is rooted, is basically a way of describing and understanding how we harmonize with our environment. It is to do with understanding how all things are ultimately striving to maintain a level of inter-dependence.

Qigong therefore directly influences our Human Qi, which permeates and animates our body and mind, by way of harmonizing the entry and exit of both Heaven and Earth Qi, and by regulating the flow of Qi within us. Astrology and various forms of divination are attempts to explain the effects of Heaven and Earth Qi upon Human Qi. Qigong is an experiential realization and manipulation of the effects of those same external forces at work within us.

Qi as "Life Force"

In terms of our health, we can consider Qi to be that factor which animates us into life. Therefore, our vitality and "aliveness" is a reflection of our level and internal distribution of Qi. If we lack Qi, or its flow is impeded in some way, then we lack vitality and may become ill. Within this narrower definition of Qi, we can equate it to our "life force." Thus, we can simply say that the difference between that which is alive and that which is not alive is the presence or absence of "aliveness," called Qi in Chinese (also Chi in Chinese and Ki in Japanese).

Western traditions view our "life force" as an esoteric phenomenon generally accepted by us as a gift from greater powers. As such, westerners have not tried to understand it to the extent that their Oriental counterparts have. The Oriental traditions see our "aliveness" and therefore our energy and vitality as much more to do with our interaction with nature's cycles.

While we are alive, Qi or "aliveness" permeates every part of our body, keeping each cell and every bodily function alive. Although cells are dying throughout our body, they are being constantly replaced. The replacement of cells declines as we get older until not enough of the essential ones required for correct organic functioning are replaced. At that time we malfunction and die. The more Qi that reaches the cells, the less prone to decay they will be, so that an abundant supply of Qi to a cell means a healthier cell. However, it is not simply a question of quantity, but also of movement. All living things exhibit more activity than their dead counterparts. Qi is flowing smoothly and abundantly in a cycle within healthy vibrant creatures. Unhealthy creatures are not vibrant, because their Qi is not flowing smoothly.

It may be that Qi is not present in adequate quantity to generate sufficient momentum to allow for a smooth flow, resulting in areas being starved of vitality while other areas stagnate and accumulate waste products; rather like insufficient water failing to flush debris from a drainage pipe. Alternatively, it may be that too much Qi is accumulating in a particular area of the body, causing stagnation or hyper-activity there. This is rather like too many cars on a constricted road, resulting in no cars moving, in turn causing potential for actual irritation and aggression (e.g., road rage in traffic jams).

So, to remain healthy or to regain health, Qi must be:

- Restored if it is deficient.

- Unblocked if it is stuck.

- Calmed if it is irritated.

- One way or another it must be kept moving.

Such imbalances in the quantity and circulation of Qi have many causes, which include the effect of emotional disturbance, shock, unbalanced mental attitude, excessive heat or cold, extreme assault from virulent organisms, poisons, poor diet, incorrect use of the body (creating postural and/or organ stress), accidents, and so on.

Qi Within Qigong

All Qigong methods aim to develop your Qi so that it can more effectively work for you. Therefore, it is worth noting that the original Chinese written character for Qi translates as "no fire." This expression at face value seems hard to understand. However, when we consider that a major goal of the Qigong practitioner is to harmonize the flow of Qi to prevent disease within the internal organs, it becomes clear. Dis-ease means the opposite of "ease" which reflects the fact that if an organ receives an improper amount of Qi (especially too much), it will become agitated, like fire, causing it to malfunction. Thus, the goal of the Qigong practitioner is to reach a state of "no fire" or ease rather than dis-ease.

The later and current written character for Qi translates as air or steam rising up from rice. This elucidates the notion that the Qi circulating in your body is enhanced by the inhalation of air and the digestion of food. Air is considered the most material form of Heaven Qi which we as humans can absorb, while the energy we get from food is the most material form of Earth Qi available to us. Qigong systems that emphasize refined breathing methods therefore aim to extract and utilize maximum Heaven Qi in the form of oxygen. Methods such as Taiji Qigong, which maintain awareness of the ground by "grounding" the feet through stance and movement, whilst encouraging regular and mindful breathing, aim to absorb both Heaven and Earth Qi. To illustrate the diversity of Qigong practice, there are also Qigong methods based around chewing food, which strongly emphasize the direct absorption of Earth Qi (in the form of Food Qi).

However, an understanding of how Qi interrelates with your mind and with your constitutional strength will help you understand how and why you should spend time building your reserves of Qi through Qigong.

■ The Three Treasures

Qi has already been discussed at some length, so you know that we must have Qi to live and more Qi to move. However, living involves a process of organic change ranging from birth and growth towards eventual decay. The underlying factor enabling birth, growth and reproduction is known as Jing (pronounced "Ching") which translates as Essence. Jing determines your constitutional strength and is the blueprint for your individual characteristics.

In western physiological terms it roughly equates to your hormonal system insofar as it is your hormones that regulate growth, reproduction, and decay and other changes in your body.* However, in traditional Daoist philosophy, the definition of Jing would encapsulate more than the physical hormonal system, although there is no need to get into such nuances here.

However, an organism can exist with sufficient Jing to fulfil the involuntary process of growth and reproduction without exhibiting an indication of consciousness. Consciousness signifies the presence of Shen, which is the energy behind the power to think and discriminate, to rationalize, and to self reflect. Without Shen there can be no personality. Qi, Jing, and Shen are known in traditional oriental thinking as the "Three Treasures" (San Bao). So in summary, we can say that everything has some degree of Qi. Only that which is "living" in the sense that it is subject to growth, reproduction and decay has Jing. Only creatures that are conscious and can self-reflect (e.g. humans) have Shen.** It is important to remember though, that Jing and Shen are limited aspects or special manifestations of Qi, as is everything else that exists. They are not really isolated in separate "boxes" and in practice, the borders between them can overlap somewhat.

How this information relates to you practicing Qigong is that the main goal of all Qigong training is to learn how to retain your Jing, strengthen and regulate your Qi flow, and illuminate your Shen.

■ More About Jing (Essence)

There are two sources of Jing or "Essence:" that acquired before birth, known as Pre-Heaven Essence, Pre-Birth Essence, or Original Essence (Yuan Jing), and that acquired after birth, called Post-Heaven Essence or Post-Birth Essence (Hou Tian Jing). Jing is a sort of concentrated Qi awaiting mobilization. In its Pre-Heaven form, it is passed onto us during conception as a union between the Jing stored in the sperm of your father and Jing

---

*Your hormonal efficiency is largely determined by the genetic characteristics passed onto you from your parents, and thereafter influenced by the way you live and the substances you ingest. Similarly, the concept of Jing is such that you have a supply inherited from your parents that is supplemented from a supply extracted from food and to some extent, air.
**That is the traditional Daoist view. It could be that other animals do have Shen. We don't really know.

stored in the ovum of your mother. In the Chinese language, sperm is called "Jing Zi," which means "Essence of the Son," because it contains the Jing passed from father to child. So once again we see the parallel between genetics and Jing. After conception, while the foetus is in the womb, it continues to receive Pre-Birth Jing from the mother through the umbilical cord. Thus, it follows that if your parents were healthy at the time of your conception, and your mother lived a healthy lifestyle throughout your time in her womb, then your Pre-Birth Essence will be strong.

Pre-Birth Essence is stored in the Kidneys and is largely fixed in quantity and quality at birth, being slowly consumed during the normal process of living, until death from old age signifies its final depletion. However, overwork, poor diet, and excessive sexual activity over a prolonged period accelerate its depletion. On the other hand, its quality can be increased and its depletion significantly slowed down through the practice of Qigong, Taiji Quan, and certain types of yoga.

The term Post-Birth Essence is given to the Jing that is extracted from food and refined by your digestive system once you have been born and thereafter throughout life. It supplements the Pre-Birth Essence, and together they form a generalized Essence that underpins the functioning of your body/mind. This generalized Essence is stored in your Kidneys, thus it is referred to as Kidney-Essence.

Interestingly, the stronger your Pre-Birth Essence, the stronger your constitution, which usually means your digestive system is stronger. This in turn means that you are naturally more efficient at extracting Post-Birth Essence from food.

Thus, Jing is rather like a powerful battery, whereas Qi is like electricity formed in that battery and which subsequently circulates to "electrify" us into activity and growth. The Pre-Birth component of your Jing is also like an inheritance of cash invested for you to get you off to a good start in life. The Post-Birth component is like the interest earned from your investment plus the money you earn from day-to-day employment. If you withdraw your monetary investment and spend it, you will have no reserves and no more interest accruing. Therefore, you will have to work harder to maintain your comforts. Similarly, if you squander your Pre-Birth Essence, you will become progressively less robust, have less resistance to disease, and you will need to take much more care about how you live and what you eat. In other words, you will have to work hard to hold onto your health.

Therefore, Jing has various functions, all concerned with growth, development, sexual maturation, and conception. It is said to fill "The Sea of Marrow," which is a generic term for the bones, brain, spinal cord, all other nerve tissue, and teeth. Your Jing therefore determines your proper growth and development and provides the basis for normal brain development.

■ Original Qi

There are several types of Qi that animate your body and mind, all basically the same but varying between more "dense" and more "rarified" in quality, and labelled according to the specific job it does. For example, one type of Qi is called Defensive Qi (Wei Qi), which is Qi in a more yang form, because it circulates quite rapidly on the exterior of your body (a yang position compared to your body's interior, which is a yin position by contrast (*see* Yin-Yang, page 32). The deepest, most fundamental manifestation of Qi in your body is known as Original Qi (Yuan Qi), which is simply Jing in a more dynamic phase. Compared to Defensive Qi, it moves more slowly and circulates at a predominately deeper level.

So, whereas Jing mostly resides in the Kidneys and circulates extremely slowly through the body, metaphorically like a viscous fluid, to provide the impetus for our physical growth, Original Qi is more energy-like and flows everywhere. However, it is still in a more fluid-like manner than Defensive Qi, which is more like a gas in the way it spreads.

Original Qi can therefore be seen as the link between Jing, which is more fluid-like and related to slow, long-term cycles and changes, and the day-to-day Qi, which is energy-like and related to short-term cycles and changes.

The importance of Jing and Original Qi to the Qigong practitioner is the crux of the practice. Qigong aims to conserve and improve the quality of the Jing stored in the Kidneys, and by so doing improve the quantity and quality of Original Qi, so that all the organs and functions of the body can be imbued with life-enhancing vitality at a deep and sustained level.

In a nutshell we can say that our level of Original Qi (Yuan Qi) in circulation directly relates to our level of vitality; so having little means we will be constantly tired and having a lot means we will have more energy to get on with life.

■ The Gate of Vitality

Your ultimate source of internal warmth and bodily functions emanates from an area deep in your abdomen, more or less between your kidneys. This area is known as the Gate of Vitality (Mingmen) within which a heating factor known as "Minister Fire" or "Life Gate Fire" transforms your Jing (Essence) into Original Qi. Within Qigong practice, the Gate of Vitality can be considered an aspect of your Lower Dantian. Focusing on and moving from your Lower Dantian during Qigong practice will naturally help keep this Life Gate Fire burning. This is a good thing because if this Fire declines, all the bodily functions will decline, causing tiredness, mental depression, and a general feeling of cold. Healthy sexual function and fertility is also dependant on the warmth of the Gate of Vitality, as is the warmth required by your digestive organs to properly break down and assimilate food.

The Lower Dantian is an area in your lower abdomen that is like a vast sea of Qi that ensures the filling of various reservoirs of Qi within your body. One way of looking at the relationship between the Gate of Vitality and the Lower Dantian is to think of the Lower Dantian as a Sea of Jing which is acted upon by the "Life Gate Fire." This causes some evaporation of that Jing into a more active, yang state, called Original Qi (Yuan Qi), which then enlivens all the organs and functions of your body via the Channels of Qi.

■ More About Shen (Mind)

Shen is usually translated as Mind or Spirit. It is your raw consciousness; in other words, the "you" which looks out at the world and wonders at it. It basically refers to your higher consciousness, so it is that "ingredient" which makes you human. Consequently, it can control other aspects of your mind, for example, by giving you the ability to override your basic instincts, rather than always succumbing to them. As a result, it gives us the faculties of free will, consideration, and contemplative thought.

In a way, it is like a control tower that directs other facets of your mind, such as your willpower, ability to plan and decide, and your capacity to think. In its role as a control tower, your Shen, through your Yi, has the power to direct your Qi to fulfil your intent.

The aspect of your mind that enables you to think with clarity and intent is called "Yi." Therefore, when doing a meditation that involves focusing your attention clearly upon a function such as your breathing, or a concept such as compassion, the success with which you can maintain clarity of thought and mental focus is dependant on the strength of your Yi. Similarly, Qigong exercises which involve you using your mind to influence a movement of Qi somewhere in your body is an example of your Yi leading your Qi.

Because your Yi is your conscious thought process, it requires a well-nourished and energized brain to manifest itself. The brain is nerve tissue, which in Chinese medicine and Qigong theory is an aspect of "marrow." The proper development of the marrow, and therefore the brain, depends upon the Kidney-Essence. Thus, it is clear that the clarity and proper functioning of your thoughts depends on the quality of your Jing.

Jing, Qi, and Shen therefore refer to three different levels of "condensation" of Qi. Jing is the most coarse and dense; Qi is more rarefied than Jing; Shen is the most subtle and immaterial. In normal living, if your Jing and Qi are depleted, your Shen will be dull. The core concept of the Three Treasures can be summarized in the following table:

Jing (vital essence)	Qi (vital energy)	Shen (mind)
Determines substance	Enables function	Creates intention
Physical body	Energy body	Consciousness

■ Enriching and Utilizing the Three Treasures Through Qigong

So, let us come back to the purpose of Qigong. We can now see from the above explanation of the Three Treasures, that it would be a good idea to look after those treasures and utilize them for maximum benefit. After all, there is no point in allowing any type of treasure to just disappear, or in hoarding it away and never benefiting from it.

The reasons for diligent Qigong practice are:

- To help protect and maintain the quality of your Jing, and thus extend the length and quality of your life.

- To strengthen your Kidneys, because that is where your Jing is rooted and stored, and from where your Original Qi emanates after its conversion from Jing (a process which takes place within the Gate of Vitality).

- To keep your Shen strong so that you can maintain sustained concentration without distraction, and thus "feel" and direct your Qi.

- To naturally encourage a more efficient circulation of Qi, which will, to a degree, result in a more efficient conversion of Original Qi from Jing, through the practice of Wai Dan (External Elixir) Qigong methods.

- At a more advanced level, to enable the practitioner to control the generation of Original Qi from Jing in a smooth, continuous stream, through Nei Dan (Internal Elixir) Qigong methods.

To summarize the importance of the Three Treasures, we should remember that Qi, Jing, and Shen are inter-dependent. When your Shen is weak, your Qi will also be weak and lack force and direction, leading to accelerated degeneration of your body. Likewise, your Qi energizes your Shen and your Jing ultimately nourishes it, so Qi and Jing keep your Shen strong and sharp. Therefore if any of the Three Treasures are weak, the others will be weakened and your whole body and mind will pay the price.

■ Channels of Qi

To further understand the essence of Qigong, you should know that Qi is flowing everywhere throughout the living body, but aggregates into "channels" of more concentrated Qi flow. As an analogy: Just as no part of your living body can be without Qi, likewise no part of a sea can be without water. Some areas of the sea will have stronger currents, resulting from the dynamic movement and interaction of the sea and of the planet as a whole. Many of these currents can be charted (such as the Gulf Stream). Likewise, within a human or animal body, the general dynamic of being alive will result in Qi aggregating along discernible courses. Over many millennia, the Chinese have mapped out these channels (or "meridians"). During that time they have noticed what happens when a channel does not flow in the way it should. Consequently, they devised ways of restoring the correct "attitude" of the channels and the Qi within them, which include all the methods of Qigong and the Oriental healing arts.

The channels run like rivers all over the surface of the body, continuing like subterranean rivers deep into the interior of the body, directing Qi into and away from all the internal organs. Where one channel begins and ends, it flows into another, so that you have a continuous circuit. Sometimes a channel will also connect with other channels elsewhere along its course. From the main or "primary" channels, stream-like branches divide off at intervals, which themselves sub-divide into more streams to supply Qi to all the bodily structures, such as muscles, fascia, bone, and so on.

The channel system is like a vast matrix supplying Qi to all areas and functions of the body, allowing interaction throughout all aspects of the body and mind, not dissimilar to the ever dividing and spreading profile of our nervous system and circulatory system.

Specifically, we have twelve pairs of **primary channels** (Jing) that, via surface and internal pathways, connect the extremities of our bodies to our internal organs, and by way of millions of tiny secondary offshoots (Luo), to all other areas of the body (Figures 2 to 13).

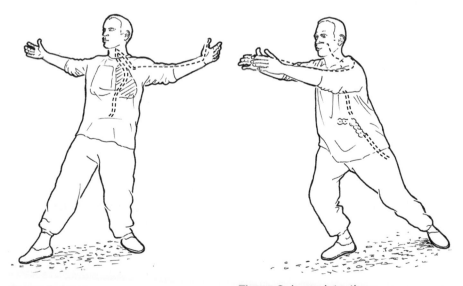

Figure 2: *Lung.*   **Figure 3:** *Large Intestine.*

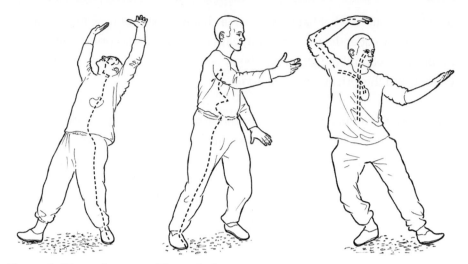

Figure 4: *Stomach.* **Figure 5:** *Spleen.* **Figure 6:** *Heart.*

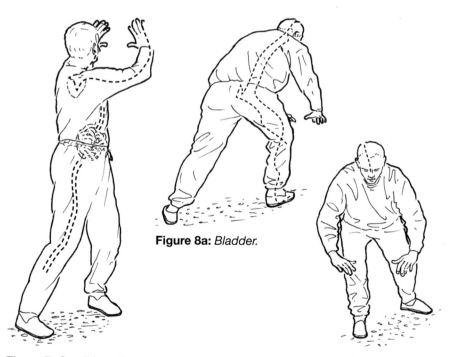

Figure 7: *Small Intestine.*

Figure 8a: *Bladder.*

Figure 8b: *Bladder.*

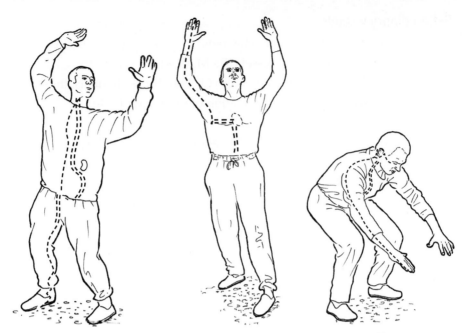

Figure 9: *Kidney.*   **Figure 10:** *Pericardium.*   **Figure 11:** *Triple Heater.*

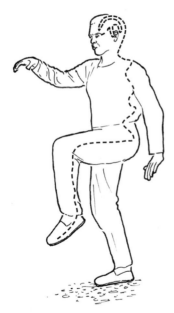

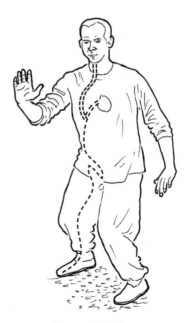

Figure 12: *Gall Bladder.*   **Figure 13:** *Liver.*

Extraordinary Vessels

In addition to the twelve primary channels, there are eight reservoirs of Qi known as extraordinary vessels (Ba Mai), which top up the Qi in the primary channels, or drain off excess Qi from those channels, thus regulating the distribution and circulation of Qi in your body.

Two of these reservoirs have particular significance within the practice of Qigong. These are the Front Mai, which runs down the vertical midline of your body on the front of your torso, and the Back Mai, which runs up the posterior midline of your body in two branches. One branch is called the *fire path* (Figure 14). This connects Ren-1 (Huiyin) to Du-1 at the base of the coccyx, then runs up the posterior border of your spinal column, over the

Baihui

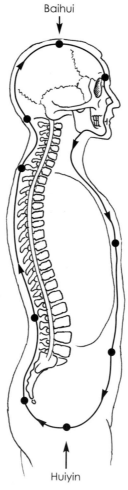

Huiyin

Figure 14: *The Fire Path Qi circulation up the Back Mai and down the Front Mai.*

midline of your cranium and down the front of your face into your palate to connect with the Front Mai, as the tongue touches the palate.

The other branch, called the *water path*, diverges from the fire path at the base of the coccyx and runs through the marrow of your spinal cord, then through your brain into the Upper Dantian, re-connecting with the *fire path* slightly anterior to Du-20 (Baihui), Figure 15.

Cultivating Qi along the *fire path* represents the basic Nei Dan practice. Conversely, developing the *water path* represents one of the deepest Nei Dan practices. There is also a direction of Qi flow that can be developed, known as the *wind path* (Figure 16). Qi flow along the wind path runs

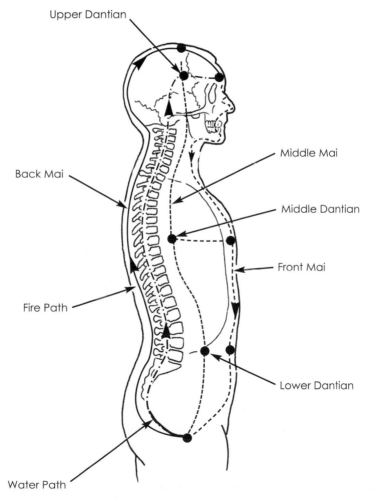

Upper Dantian
Back Mai
Fire Path
Water Path
Middle Mai
Middle Dantian
Front Mai
Lower Dantian

Figure 15: *Front Mai, Back Mai, and Middle Mai, including the Fire Path and Water Path.*

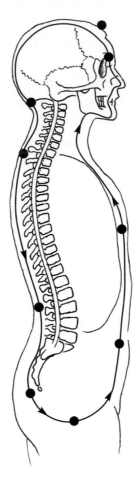

Figure 16: *The Wind Path Qi circulation up the Front Mai and Down the Back Mai.*

up the Front Mai and down the Back Mai, i.e., in precisely the opposite direction to the *fire path*. Cultivating Qi flow along the *wind path* is not such a common practice as encouraging Qi to flow along the *fire path*.

The Front Mai is approximately equivalent to what in Chinese medicine is called the Ren Mai or Conception Vessel (or Directing Vessel). The Back Mai is approximately equivalent to the Du Mai or Governing Vessel. However, for the purposes of Qigong practice and theory, it is better to use the terms Front Mai and Back Mai to avoid confusion, because the Back Mai contains aspects of the Ren Mai's deep pathway, and the Front Mai contains aspects of the Du Mai's deep pathway. In reality it is all linked together, so the different terminology merely reflects differences in the way these Qi pathways are mapped out for the sake of labelling. Hence, the division and therefore the labelling is slightly different within the context of Qigong compared to that for acupuncture.

As a Qigong practitioner, another important vessel or Mai to be aware of is the Middle Mai. This, for the purpose of Qigong practice, can be simply experienced and visualized as a vertical route of Qi through the center of your torso and head, just in front of your spine, linking the Lower, Middle, and Upper Dantians. Within sitting Nei Dan practice, the Middle Mai can actually be experienced as Qi that moves vertically upward from the Lower Dantian to just above the head, and moves downward from the Lower Dantian to Ren-1 (Huiyin). Some practitioners experience it as a sky-blue light.

Note that the Middle Mai is depicted in many Qigong diagrams as the Chong Mai or Penetrating Vessel. However, the Chong Mai has deep pathways through the spinal cord and elsewhere which can cause confusion with the Front Mai and Back Mai, hence it lends clarity to call it the Middle Mai in this context.

■ Dantian

There are areas within the head and torso which are pierced centrally by the Middle Mai and intersect with the Front Mai and Back Mai which have especially abundant Qi, and are collectively known as Dantian or "Seas of Qi." Dantian literally translates as "Elixir Field," so named because the quality and level of Qi that resides within these areas are considered the key to a long and healthy life. The Elixir Fields can therefore be thought of as oceans that supply the reservoirs (Extraordinary Vessels). The purpose of Qigong is to add more Qi to these Elixir Fields so that you can have a virtually unlimited resource of Qi for the purpose of extending your life as the most vibrant person possible in order to achieve your highest goals.

By far the most important of the three Dantians (Figure 17) is the Lower Dantian (Xia Dantian). The front "shore" of this "sea" or "field" is situated behind Ren-4 (Guanyuan) and Ren-6 (Qihai), specifically about 1¾ in. (4 cm) below your umbilicus and about 1¾ in. (4 cm) deep. Remember that Dantian is a "sea" of Qi, so you shouldn't think of it as just a small point in the body. However, the epicenter of this lower sea is the center of your energy from a number of perspectives, as will become clear from reading

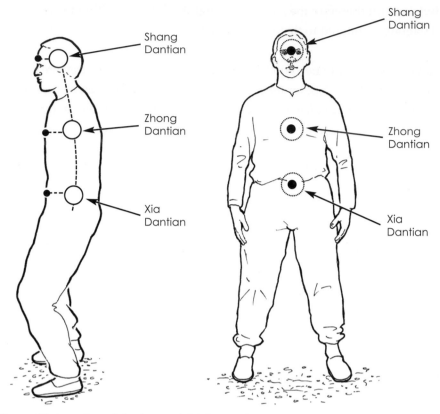

Figure 17: *Location of the Lower, Middle, and Upper Dantian.*

through this book. For now, remember it as that area where you focus your mind whenever you want to "center" your thoughts, emotions, and postural balance. It is also the point from which all efficient movements are rooted and pivot around. Therefore, the physical movements and the mental focus within Taiji Qigong use the Lower Dantian as an anchor. A sort of base to move out from and to come back to.

The other two Dantians are the Middle Dantian (Zhong Dantian) situated within the center of your chest, and the Upper Dantian (Shang Dantian) situated in the region of your forehead within the frontal lobes of your brain.

NOTE: *It is important not to get chilled around your lower abdomen, which includes the Lower Dantian and your lower back. This is because the source of warmth and therefore of activity for your entire body emanates from the Gate of Vitality; that area deep in your abdomen, more or less* *between your kidneys (see page 18). If practicing Qigong outside, make sure your lower belly and lower back do not get exposed to a chilly draught.*

■ Energy Points or "Qi Vortices" Along the Qi Channels

At specific locations along the Qi channels there are "gateways" or "cavities" (translated from Xue in Chinese, or Tsubo in Japanese) where Qi can open to the surface (Figure 18). These cavities are essentially points where Qi can:

a) Enter the channel from outside the body;

b) Leave the channel to connect with the outside world; or

c) Represent distortions in the channel flow, so that when "activated" (for example by pressure, needles, or in the case of Qigong, by focusing the mind with unwavering attention upon them) can affect the channel and therefore affect specific aspects of our body/mind function.

Some cavities do all of the above, whilst others only do one or two.

A cavity is a vortex of Qi that, if you could see it, would look like a vase-shaped swirl of energy with a mouth leading into a narrower neck, widening into a broader belly. The word "cavity" depicts a rather dead space, but these vortices are very much "alive." For that reason, I prefer to call them "Qi vortices."

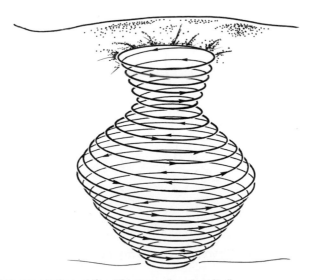

Figure 18: *Representation of the "Qi vortex" or "cavity."*

Each of the primary channels of Qi has a number of "fixed" Qi vortices. Centuries of documented observation have resulted in each Qi vortex being given a name, number, and recognized action on the body and mind when stimulated; either through acupuncture, acupressure, Qigong massage, or Qigong mental focus.

Some commonly used Qi vortices can be utilized within some of the 18 Stances of Taiji Qigong (Figures 19 & 20).

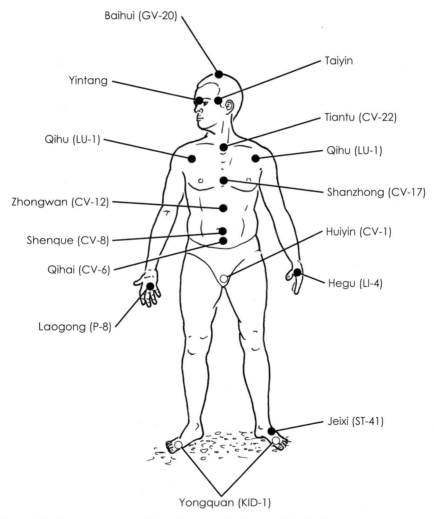

Figure 19: *Some important Qi vortices on the front of the body.*

In addition to the fixed Qi vortices, there are "transient cavity vortices" which come and go along the channels between the fixed Qi vortices. Hence, due to their impermanence, they have no names or numbers. They arise where and when they do because there is either a lack of Qi or an excessive build up of Qi at that location and at that point in time along the channel. Bodywork systems such as Shiatsu specifically focus on re-balancing these transient Qi vortices. Regular Qigong practice will also naturally smooth the flow of Qi throughout your body and so discourage extremes of hyper- or hypo-Qi concentrations at those points.

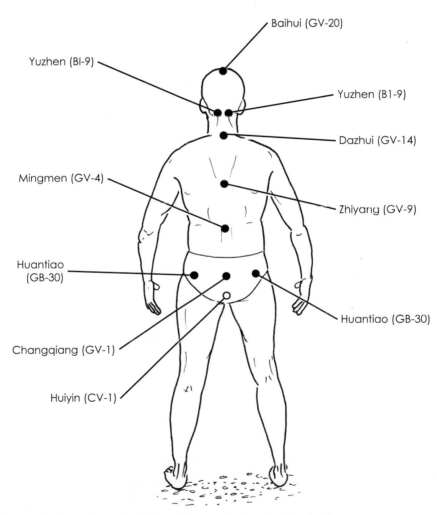

Figure 20: *Some important Qi vortices on the back of the body.*

■ Yin and Yang

As stated before, Qi is the factor that activates the universe and all within it, including ourselves. When operating within us, it acts rather like the way electricity powers a machine. To further understand how Qi behaves, it is important to have a basic understanding of Yin-Yang theory.

Yin-Yang theory is an ancient Chinese conceptual framework within the Daoist philosophy that serves as a means for viewing and understanding the world. It is the foundation for understanding all phenomena and, in the context of Chinese medicine and Qigong, for understanding health and disease.

Think of the Dao as the latent universe, before it has manifested itself. A sort of total integration that is all-encompassing, so there is nothing to compare and contrast it with; hence it cannot be perceived with our senses. Yin-Yang is the duality that manifests out of the Dao. In other words, it polarizes the Universe (Dao) into opposing phenomena that we can perceive. For example, we could not perceive light if we had no experience and concept of dark, and vice versa. We could not grasp the idea of "up" if we had no concept of "down," and so on. In other words, Yin-Yang are inseparable from the Dao, yet they are the two hands through which the Dao manifests and orders creation.

The ultimate aim of those who practice Qigong as a tool to gain spiritual insight is to shift their awareness beyond the everyday, familiar duality of Yin-Yang, to reach a perception of "emptiness," or the state of neutrality before or between Yin-Yang. This state is called Wuji. When you experience Wuji, you experience a universe where there is no subject or object, just a continuum where everything is part of everything else. Wuji is symbolized by an empty circle (Figure 21).

The ultimate Qigong or Taiji practitioner is able to move their perception between the reality of duality (Yin-Yang) and of "no extremes" (Wuji) at will. In Western philosophy, contrary ideas oppose each other. Take day and night: if it is day it cannot be night. Logically, propositions that contradict one another must oppose one another. But in the Chinese model, Yin and Yang oppose and *complement* one another. Yin and Yang are contrary, but they can turn into one another and they each contain a small part of the other.

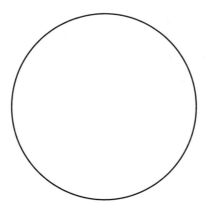

Figure 21: *The empty circle symbol of Wuji.*

Yin-Yang theory was developed during the Yin and Chou dynasties, i.e., between 1500 and 221 BC. The first mention of them in a text is around 800 BC in the Yi Jing (or I Ching), the Book of Changes, and it is the aspect of change and of process that is at the heart of Yin-Yang theory. The characters for Yin and Yang are, respectively:

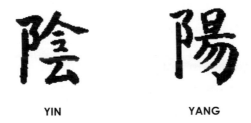

YIN   **YANG**

Putting the different components of the characters together, Yin is the cloudy or shady side of the hill and Yang the sunny side. On the Yang side it is light, warm and people are working while on the shady side it is cold, dark and everyone is resting (Figure 22).

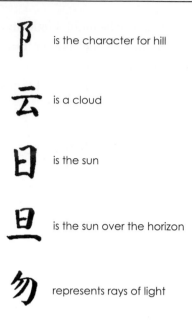

阝 is the character for hill

云 is a cloud

日 is the sun

旦 is the sun over the horizon

勿 represents rays of light

Seen in this way Yin and Yang are opposing qualities:

	In the Yin category	In the Yang category
	Darkness	Light
	Cold	Heat
	Rest	Movement
Also:	Moon	Sun
	Earth	Heaven
	West (sun sets)	East (sun rises)
	North	South

It is not, however, that Yin and Yang simply sort phenomena into fixed categories. They are a way of explaining dynamic processes. **Yin and Yang are relative terms**. Something is Yin (or Yang) only in relation to something else. So a 100-watt light bulb is more Yang than a 30- watt bulb, but it is more Yin than the sun. To say that an apple, for instance, is Yin is incorrect. It may be Yin (that is colder) in relation to a steaming bowl of soup, or it may be Yang (that is warmer) in relation to a tub of ice cream.

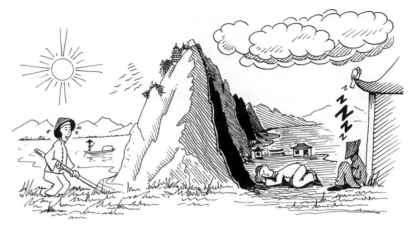

Figure 22: *Yin-Yang characterized by the sunny and shady sides of a hill.*

It doesn't make sense to talk of Yin except in relation to Yang; they are opposing but also complementary. The two make up the full picture, without one the other is incomplete. Take the Taiji symbol, the symbol of Yin-Yang (Figure 23).

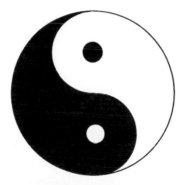

Figure 23: *Taiji: the Yin-Yang symbol.*

Yang is the white part of the symbol and Yin is the black part of the symbol. The two components coil around each other, they penetrate each other, they fade into one another. They are opposites yet they complement one another. The white part of the symbol contains a black spot and the black part a white spot: nothing is ever entirely Yin or Yang but each contains something of the other, which may grow so that eventually each can become its opposite.

Yin and Yang phenomena can themselves be further divided into Yin and Yang. For example, day is Yang compared to night, but a day may be divided into morning and afternoon. Morning, when the sun is rising, is more Yang than the afternoon, when the sun is setting, so morning is Yang and afternoon is Yin. Morning turns into afternoon, and in the same way Yang turns into Yin, and Yin into Yang. Day becomes night, summer turns to winter, our bodies move then rest, we are warm then cool, we wake and then sleep. The movement from Yin to Yang is therefore cyclical.

Another way of looking at Yin and Yang is to regard them as different states or stages of being. In the course of the cyclical movement from Yang to Yin and back again, matter takes on different forms. It is trans-formed. For example: day turns to night and during the day the sun evaporates water from the earth and seas, forming vapour which condenses as evening approaches and is precipitated as dew during the cool of the night. That which evaporates, rises, and is less substantial or formless, is Yang in relation to that which condenses, falls downward, is substantial and has form, which is Yin. To take this a little further, that which is non-material, more refined, less tangible, energetic rather than solid, is Yang in relation to what is solid, material, more gross and tangible, which is Yin.

Returning to the Yin-Yang categories of earlier, and remembering that these are **RELATIVE** qualities, we can add to the list:

YIN	YANG
Matter/substance	Energy/thought
Solid/liquid	Vapour/gas
Condensation	Evaporation
Contraction	Expansion
Descending	Rising
Below	Above
Form	Activity
Water	Fire
Yielding	Resistant
Soft	Hard
Passive	Aggressive
Introverted	Outgoing

	Quiet	Loud
	Slow	Fast
	Wet	Dry
	Chronic	Acute
Anatomy	Lower part (body)	Upper part (head)
	Interior (internal organs)	Exterior (skin, muscles)
	Medial (Yin channels)	Lateral (Yang channels)
	Front (Yin channels)	Back (Yang channels)
Physiology	Store vital substances	Digest and excrete
	Substance	Activity
	Blood and body fluids	Qi
	Down-bearing	Upward-moving
	Inward movement	Outward movement
	Yin moves energy …	Yang moves energy …
	(… and substances) down to anus and urethra	(… and substances) out to skin and limbs

There are five main ways in which Yin and Yang are related to one another.

1. Yin and Yang are Opposites

Yin and Yang struggle against one another and keep the other in check.
Cold cools down heat: cooling drinks refresh on a hot day. Heat warms up
cold: a fire heats you up on a cold day.

This is the basis of treatment in Oriental medicine: if you have a hot
condition, treatment should be cooling, and vice versa. Treatment opposes
one force with a contrary one. Likewise, in the deeper Internal Elixir
(Nei Dan) Qigong methods, Qi begins to radically move, so excessive heat
can build up in the body if the Qi flow is restricted in any way. Hence,
various practices are included which are specifically cooling.

The struggle between Yin and Yang results in a state of dynamic balance,
i.e., a balance that involves constant change rather than a fixed stasis.
In the body as in other spheres, the balance is constantly changing.
Take body temperature for example: it is basically stable, but within a

certain narrow range, it fluctuates. If it fluctuates beyond that particular range, the physiological balance of the body is lost and disease arises.

2. Yin and Yang are Interdependent

Going back to the Taiji symbol, out of Yang comes Yin, out of Yin comes Yang. Without the one the other cannot come into being. Without Yang there would be no production of Yin; without Yin there would be no production of Yang. Each promotes the other, each brings the other into being.

3. Yin and Yang Tend to Consume One Another

This means that where Yin predominates, it will overwhelm and use up Yang, and vice versa. For the body to work normally and keep itself warm (Yang), it has to burn up part of its substance (Yin). On the other hand, producing nutrient substances for the body (Yin) consumes a bit of energy (Yang). If either the Yin or Yang aspects of the body go beyond the normal range, the result is either an excess or a deficiency of them; resulting in disease.

4. Yin and Yang can Transform into One Another

The cycle of day receding into night and of night receding into day is an example of this. The annual cycle of the seasons is another example.

5. Yin and Yang can be Further Divided into Yin and Yang

I gave the example earlier about day dividing further into morning and afternoon. Likewise one can divide the year into summer (Yang) and winter (Yin), or further into summer (Yang within Yang), autumn (Yin within (coming out of) Yang), winter (Yin within Yin) and spring (Yang within (coming out of) Yin).

Furthermore, Yin and Yang are infinitely divisible.

■ What Does Qigong Really Mean?

Qigong is a word and concept from China. The broad and correct meaning of Qigong is; *any training or study dealing with Qi which takes a long time and great effort to master*. In that sense, even shiatsu and acupuncture are forms of Qigong. However, in modern use, it has come to mean; *practices that encourage Qi development and harmony within the body*.

External and Internal Elixir Categories

There are hundreds of Qigong methods, each with many variations. Each method can be grouped into one of two distinct categories: External Elixir (Wai Dan) and Internal Elixir (Nei Dan).

When practicing External Elixir methods (Wai Dan), Qi builds up in your arms and legs because you focus your attention on your limbs. This "attention" can range from consciously tensing the muscles of the limbs, which is a characteristic of many of the martial-based Qigong methods, to simply feeling the movement of your limbs brush through the air as you move. The latter is a method more characteristic of Wai Dan methods, which emphasize self-healing or the healing of others.

When the Qi in your limbs reaches a high level, it washes through the channels, clearing away obstructions to eventually nourish your internal organs. Up to a point, any physical activity achieves this, which you'll know from your experience of feeling healthier when you exercise your whole body, compared to how you feel when you sit around for long periods. Wai Dan theory is therefore based on the idea of keeping the flow of Qi strong and smooth within your Primary and Connecting Channels (Jing Luo), so that it nourishes your internal organs and functions via those channels (Figure 24). Any surplus Qi resulting from your efforts naturally accumulates in the reservoirs of Qi known as Extraordinary Vessels.

By contrast, during the practice of Internal Elixir methods (Nei Dan), Qi builds up deep within the body and is led outward into the limbs. Nei Dan methods are considered "deeper" because they are more difficult to practice, and when fully mastered bestow greater benefits and control of Qi. They have traditionally been kept more hidden than External methods; usually being taught only to select disciples within closed circles. This is because Nei Dan is more difficult to understand, dangerous to the practitioner if they get it wrong, and requires very close personal supervision to recognize the correct sensations that mark progress. At its deeper levels, Nei Dan requires a level of time and restraint that few people are able to commit to. It requires a high degree of sexual abstinence to conserve your Essence (see page 15) and freedom from distraction to practice full time. So unless you can, a) find a remote place in the mountains with food and shelter, b) are prepared to forget about having sex for a long time, and c) happen to have a Qigong master available and willing to guide you through the training, then your chances of mastering Nei Dan at a deep level (i.e., without killing yourself or going mad) are slim.

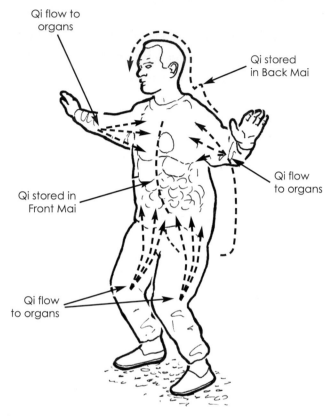

Qi flow to organs

Qi stored in Back Mai

Qi flow to organs

Qi stored in Front Mai

Qi flow to organs

Figure 24: *Qi flowing from limbs to internal organs and surplus Qi flowing into Front and Back Mai.*

However, some of the elementary and less intense methods of Nei Dan can be practiced within everyday life, although only a certain level of achievement can be reached this way. Nevertheless, such levels of achievement are well worth the effort for those willing to learn them correctly and with patience.

Theories pertaining to Nei Dan are explained in some books dealing specifically with Nei Dan practice. If you want to practice the deeper Nei Dan methods, find a suitable and qualified teacher first. Unfortunately, there aren't many of them around, especially those who have the time to teach others, given that serious Nei Dan practice is more or less a full time occupation in itself.

To summarize, it can be said that Wai Dan practice is mostly physical and generates Qi in the limbs, which then flows into the organs and slightly into the Front Mai and Back Mai, which ultimately link with the Middle Mai. Nei Dan practice is mostly mental and generates Qi in the body, mainly within the Front Mai, Back Mai, Middle Mai, and the organs, then spreads it to the limbs, skin, and marrow.

Note that bodywork healing systems based on Qi, such as acupuncture, shiatsu, and tuina are essentially akin to Wai Dan Qigong methodology insofar as they manipulate Qi via techniques applied to the exterior of the body.

Passive and Active Methods

External and Internal Qigongs can further be divided into Passive (Jing Gong) and Active (Dong Gong) methods.

Passive Qigongs are meditative practices that emphasize stillness, awareness of internal movements, and "attitudes" of Qi, plus some internal visualizations. These can be done while sitting, lying, or standing. Passive Qigongs are predominantly used for Internal Elixir (Nei Dan) methods, although not exclusively.

Active Qigongs emphasize slow movement, with or without specific methods of breathing. They can be used as a vehicle for either Internal or External Elixir (Wai Dan) methods.

There is also a third category involving sudden spontaneous movements arising out of a static stance. All methods are designed to reap long-term benefits resulting from long-term practice, rather than as a quick way to feel good.

Qigong Categories According to One's Aspirations

We can also classify all Qigongs, whether Internal, External, Active, or Passive, into four categories according to the aspirations of the practitioner. These categories are:

1. Personal health and longevity;

2. Medical Qigong for healing others;

3. Martial skill;

4. Enlightenment.

However, most Qigongs exist under more than one of these headings; for example, they all tend to increase personal vitality, plus generate a level of "insight" purely through the intense focus of the practice.

Where Does 18-Stance Taiji Qigong Fit In?

Taiji Qigong is based on a continuous flow of slowly executed movements which of themselves give positive health benefits. However, if done mindfully, with some internal awareness or "feeling" of Qi, plus some visualizations, the effects are enhanced. In that sense, Taiji Qigong can be considered a form of meditation in movement. Many of the movements are taken from Taiji Quan (Tai ch'i), which is essentially a martial art. Some of these Taiji Quan movements have been modified within Taiji Qigong to amplify their therapeutic effect at the expense of their martial application.

The 18 Stances of Taiji Qigong are commonly practiced as an Active External Elixir method. That is, you make slow movements to generate Qi in the limbs. During these movements, you fix your attention on any sensations you feel in those limbs. During many of the exercises, you imagine the moving limbs are subject to some form of subtle resistance. For example, if moving your arms forwards, you imagine you are pushing something away from you. Alternatively, you can imagine the resistance comes from you visualizing yourself doing the exercises within a substance slightly more viscous than water, such as heavy oil. This enhanced Qi within your limbs is then automatically directed into your body to rejuvenate your organs. It can also be directed back out through your hands to facilitate healing through bodywork.

Taiji Qigong can also be practiced as a deep Internal Elixir method, but that is outside the scope of this book. However, some of the exercises lend themselves to a variety of simple internal visualizations and techniques that are safe and easy to learn from a book such as this. Examples of such visualizations and techniques will be given with some of the exercises where applicable. For now, an understanding of the movement of Qi through the Front Mai and Back Mai vessels, as described below under "The Small Circulation," will clarify the reasons for some of the instructions given.

■ The Small Circulation

At the level of Taiji Qigong practice, some Nei Dan preparatory practices can be employed to open up the Small Circulation (Xiao Zhou Tian), sometimes called Lesser Heavenly Circuit or Microcosmic Orbit (Figure 25). This circuit is formed by the joining of the Front Mai and the Back Mai.

The method for preparing the opening of the Small Circulation is to increase Qi in the Lower Dantian through abdominal breathing or by simply focusing your mind on your lower abdomen (*see* page 60).

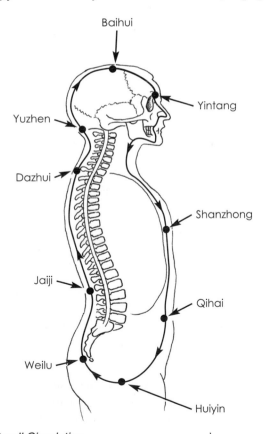

Figure 25: *The Small Circulation.*

When Qi is sufficiently abundant in the Lower Dantian, the practitioner uses his mind to lead the Qi down from Dantian to Huiyin (Ren-1) and then to the tailbone (Du-1). From Du-1, the Qi is led up the back of the spine, over the crown of the head, and down the front of the body, back to the Lower Dantian to complete the cycle. This circuit is the way Qi naturally circulates in a healthy person.

If the Small Circulation is visualized in Taiji Qigong (or better still, "experienced"), it is done to gently encourage the natural circulation of Qi within that circuit, often as a preparation for deeper Nei Dan practices in the future.

When incorporated in the Nei Dan practices, leading the Qi through this circuit is done in a more prolonged and intensely focused way, and requires the opening of the various "gates" within the circuit, before Qi can safely be accumulated there. The three main gates through which it is most difficult to circulate Qi are:

1. Weilu (in the region of Du-1: Changqiang);

2. Jiaji (in the region of Du-4: Mingmen);

3. Yuzhen (Bladder-9: Yuzhen).***

This practice can therefore be done within passive sitting or standing Qigong or incorporated into some of the Taiji Qigong exercises. A higher Nei Dan practice is to then lead the Qi to the extremities and to the skin and bone marrow.

The ability to do this is called Grand Circulation (Da Zhou Tian), also known as the Greater Heavenly Circuit, the details of which are outside the necessity and scope of this book.

***Although Bl-9 is not directly on the Back Mai, but about ¾ in. (2 cm) lateral to it, this reflects the fact that Qi spreads a little as it goes over the head. If it spreads too much, it will interfere with the normal brain function. Therefore, it must be contained within the lateral parameters defined by Bladder-9.

PART II

General Principles of Qigong Practice

■ How Much Should You Practice?

The benefits that can be attained from Qigong are proportional to the amount you practice. Fifteen minutes a day is time well spent. If you can work up to and maintain a regular 30 minute session twice a day, you will notice a marked increase in vitality and serenity within one month. If you can work up to a couple of hours every day, there will very soon be a radical improvement in your health and level of Qi. If you are healthy when you start you will become healthier, and if you are ill when you start you will begin to feel better (if you really do it! There is a difference between just going through the motions to "get it done" and really focusing your practice).

At any given time you can either practice the full set of eighteen movements, or pick and choose the one's you like best. Sometimes the one's you like are the one's you need most to maintain your Qi levels. On the other hand, if you are doing Qigong to combat a chronic illness, it is a good idea to practice some movements that have less immediate appeal to you. This is because your problem may be reflected in a blockage of Qi, which makes those particular Qigong movements slightly uncomfortable or tedious. Persevering with those movements with mindfulness and patience will eventually restore the free flow of Qi within the affected region.

There is no set rule to how many repetitions of each movement you should perform. However, for many people in China, the standard for Taiji Qigong is six repetitions or multiples of six. Others traditionally like to stick to odd numbers for most things. Hence, three or five repetitions are common.

■ Optimum Conditions for Practice

Time of Day to Practice

You can practice Qigong any time of day (or night!). As dawn breaks and at dusk are especially good times because there is a natural calmness in the air at that time. This is because the energies of day (more Yang) and night (more Yin) are equally balanced as night slowly turns into day and day gradually recedes into night. This effect is obviously much more marked in a rural setting.

Which Direction to Face

Many practitioners like to face the sun in the early morning, because it is felt that much Heaven Qi can be absorbed from the sun as it rises. In the evening it is considered beneficial to face south (or north if in the southern hemisphere), because it is believed that the Qi within you aligns itself with the earth's magnetic field, to allow a greater absorption of Earth Qi. In the middle of the day your direction is not so important. Personally, if I am located such that I can feel the direct warmth of the sun, I sometimes prefer to face directly into that warmth, or occasionally I like to feel the warmth on my back.

However, if I happen to be on the edge of the seashore or overlooking an open view from a height, facing straight out to the horizon seems more powerful and relevant than the position of the sun. If you are indoors, facing the light from a window usually feels best.

With practice, your sensitivity to such things will grow and you will naturally position yourself to face the most appropriate direction, which will in fact be the predominant source of energy.

Another traditional view is to take into consideration the directions which relate to certain internal Organs:

- Facing East may help strengthen a weak Liver.

- Facing West may help sedate an overactive Liver.

- Facing West may help strengthen weak Lungs.

- Facing East may help sedate tight and congested Lungs.

- Facing North may help strengthen weak Kidneys.

- Facing South may help strengthen a weak Heart.

Again, I would say that any direction that feels right will be more effective for you than choosing a direction according to the theory. If you are not sensitive to such things at the moment, experimenting with the directions according to tradition or theory is actually a good way of acquiring that sensitivity.

Where to Practice

Qigong can be practiced almost anywhere, but some places are better than others. The best places are where the Heaven and Earth Qi are most abundant, and the frenetic hussle and bussle of "civilization" is absent. If you should find yourself high in the mountains next to a waterfall in pleasantly warm weather, then that would be ideal. The seashore is also excellent because moving water generates lots of Qi. The mountains or seashore also has the advantage of being relatively free from atmospheric pollution.

If you don't happen to be in the mountains or by the sea, at least try to stay well away from traffic fumes, excessive noise, and the electromagnetic radiation from TV sets, computers, etc. Try to find a quiet and peaceful space indoors or outdoors with plenty of fresh air, but avoiding draughts.

What to Wear

Wear loose comfortable clothing, ideally made of natural fibers, and remove watches and bracelets because they constrict the Qi flowing through the wrist. Also, because you wear one watch on one wrist, there will be a sense of asymmetry when you raise your arms. If you insist on wearing such jewellery, put the watch on one wrist and the bracelet(s) on the other to at least get some symmetry of weight distribution. It may not seem significant from just reading this, but when your sensitivity grows through practice, you will really feel like the watch is in the way.

Feeling too cold during your session will dramatically reduce the sensations and benefits you might otherwise experience. If it is chilly, dress appropriately. It is especially important to wear warm gloves if you have cold hands. Once you are well established in your practice, your hands will begin to warm up immediately or very soon after you begin your Qigong routine. Keep your belly and back warm as well, because chilling your Lower Dantian and kidneys will severely restrict your Qi circulation, which is the exact opposite of what you are trying to do through the practice of Qigong.

Menstruation and Pregnancy

It is good to practice basic Qigong during menstruation or pregnancy, because it will improve circulation of Qi, blood, and the other body fluids. However, avoid the more advanced methods and stick to natural breathing. Also, if you have a very heavy period, it is better to focus on the center of the chest (Shanzhong: Ren-17), rather than Dantian in the lower belly, because focusing on Dantian may increase the flow still further.

Pregnancy should give you a heightened awareness of your belly and of your "earthiness." Qigong also gives you a heightened awareness of your belly and grounds you. Therefore, pregnancy could be an opportunity to naturally improve your Qigong. Practicing Qigong during pregnancy is also an excellent opportunity to "connect" with your unborn child through that belly-centered focus.

Other Considerations

If you are at home with plenty of time and about to embark upon a serious session of at least half an hour, it can be useful to have a quick brisk shower, followed by a brisk drying off with the towel. This will in itself freshen up your Qi. However, you should never feel that doing Qigong is a hassle, so the shower is not crucial; it's just an extra ingredient, and it would be silly to skip your Qigong session just because you didn't feel like showering.

Being distracted by hunger will not help your mental focus and determination, so if you are hungry, eat something light. Don't practice straight after a heavy meal because your Qi will be diverted into your digestive system, leaving very little to circulate elsewhere. Particularly avoid alcohol if you are about to practice: this will make you feel tired, weak, maybe dizzy, or even sick. If you get distracted and feel you should stop your session, close with the Balancing Qi movement (Movement 18— *see* page 144).

■ Correct Posture and Stance to Begin

Although Taiji Qigong is an active method of Qigong, the starting position is in itself a passive Qigong aimed at opening the flow of Qi and centering your mind. The important thing is to hold your spine in vertical alignment between your pelvis and head to get maximum polarity between Heaven Qi and Earth Qi, so that maximum Heaven Qi and Earth Qi is attracted into your body. Specifically, you should make sure that the point called Huiyin (Ren-1, DV-1, or CV-1) which is situated between your legs and midway between your anus and genitals, is in vertical alignment with Baihui (Du-20 or GV-20), situated on top of your head in a line between the apex of your ears (Figure 26). Huiyin is used in many Qigong exercises as a point to contain and gather the Yin energies of the body, whereas Baihui is considered the most Yang point of the body and therefore the opposite in location and function to Huiyin.

Also, in the beginning stance, and any stance where the feet are parallel and between hip-width and shoulder-width apart, the alignment between Baihui and Huiyin should extend down to a line level with a point on top of each foot called Jeixi (Stomach-41). This lies in a depression between the two prominent tendons on the front of your ankle joint (Figure 26).

If you lose this vertical alignment by bending forward, you will inhibit the ability of your lungs to inhale efficiently, thus denying yourself optimum oxygen/Qi uptake from the air.

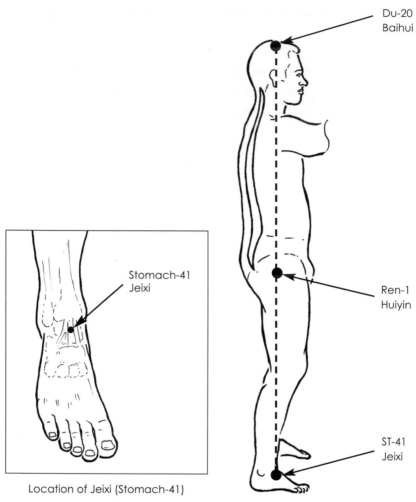

Du-20
Baihui

Stomach-41
Jeixi

Ren-1
Huiyin

ST-41
Jeixi

Location of Jeixi (Stomach-41)

Figure 26: *Postural alignment through Baihui, Huiyin, and Jeixi points.*

If you bend backward, you will compress your spinal joints and so block the flow of Qi along your spine, losing the polarity and connection between Heaven Qi and Earth Qi within your body. In fact your spinal joints should be encouraged to "open" as much as possible to get maximum distance between your head and pelvis, thus maintaining maximum length in your spinal column. This is because Qi flows much more easily through joints that move freely and have space within them compared to those that are stiff and contracted.

Paradoxically, consciously pushing your head and pelvis in opposite directions will merely contract your postural muscles and shorten your spine. Lengthening and true alignment of the spine can only be achieved through relaxation and mental focus. If you remember to frequently check your alignment, relaxation, and mental focus during any of the movements and positions, you will steadily progress.

In this basic starting position, you can benefit from reflecting upon the melding of Heaven Qi and Earth Qi within you as a human being, where the downward flow of Heaven Qi meets the upward flow of Earth Qi.

Regarding the position of your feet in the basic standing position, it is best to keep them as near parallel to each other as possible. Here, parallel means that the big toes should be the same distance apart as the heels.

If the toes are closer together than the heels, the point in your lower back called Mingmen (GV-4) will be too open, causing a loss of energy through that "gate" (Figure 27). If the toes are too wide in relation to the heels, the Mingmen will remain closed, preventing Qi flowing up the Back Mai (Figure 28).

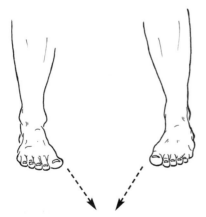

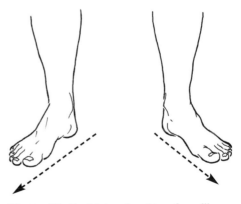

Figure 27: *Feet turned in too far will cause leakage of Qi from Mingmen.*

Figure 28: *Feet turned out too far will cause blockage of Qi at Mingmen, and consequent restriction of Qi flow up the Back Mai.*

For Taiji Qigong and most other Qigong methods done in the standing position, the basic starting position (Figure 29a & b) is described below:

- Stand with your feet parallel, placed between hip-width and shoulder-width apart or slightly wider if that's more comfortable: as if a large imaginary ball situated between your knees is stopping them from drifting together.

- Keep your knees slightly bent; just enough to "unlock" them. Don't allow the knees to extend beyond the toes.

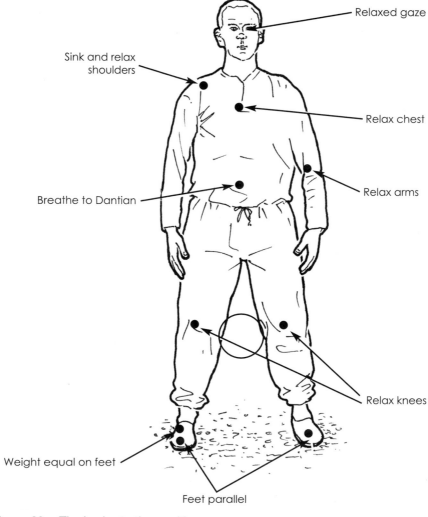

Figure 29a: *The basic starting position.*

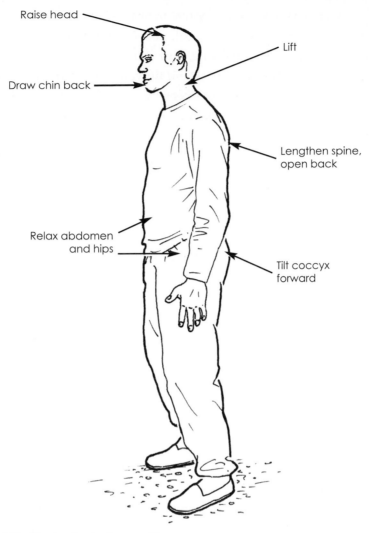

Raise head

Lift

Draw chin back

Lengthen spine, open back

Relax abdomen and hips

Tilt coccyx forward

Figure 29b: *The basic starting position.*

- Initially, feel that your weight is evenly distributed between your heels and the balls of your feet.

- If you are outside standing at a high point, fix your eyes on the horizon. If you are indoors, or with no view of a far horizon, look forward and slightly downward. If you are a complete beginner, it is recommended that you keep your eyes shut during the first few weeks of practice, so that you can direct all your attention inward without distraction.

- If your eyes are open, keep them very relaxed, not wide open or closed, but somewhere in between. This is synonymous with a relaxed demeanour, where you are receptive to feeling subtle sensations and where your attention will most easily relate to the present. Release all tension in your neck, allowing your chin to drop very slightly as you gently hold your throat back and lift your occiput from your atlas vertebra. This will lengthen your neck by naturally lifting your head up; almost like an Edwardian gentleman raising his top hat as a gesture of courtesy.

- Drop your shoulders and elbows so that your arms hang loosely by your side. Your shoulders should not be down and back, military style, but down and slightly forward. This will allow your chest to relax and your belly to feel and look more "open." Note that this does not mean you should collapse or depress the chest, rather that you should feel the ribs softening and spreading, with a sense of opening downward.

- Relax your hips and abdomen with your spine in natural alignment with the top of your head.

- Now visualize your pelvis as a bowl of water positioned between your legs and lower torso. Centrally position your "bowl" so that it is not tilted forward or backward (imagining that you are trying not to spill any water out of the bowl). Hence, your coccyx should naturally tilt slightly forward under your torso. This will have the effect of straightening your lumbar spine.

- The effect of implementing the above instructions will be that the Qi will become unlocked from your upper body and collect in your Lower Dantian, which is the reservoir of Qi in your lower abdomen.

■ Refining Your Stance

After a few weeks of regular practice, or when you feel ready, you can begin to include additional factors and visualizations to increase the effectiveness of your stance (Figure 30).

- Focus your mind on Kidney-1 in both feet. Kidney-1 (Yongquan) is a point just behind the center of the ball of the foot.

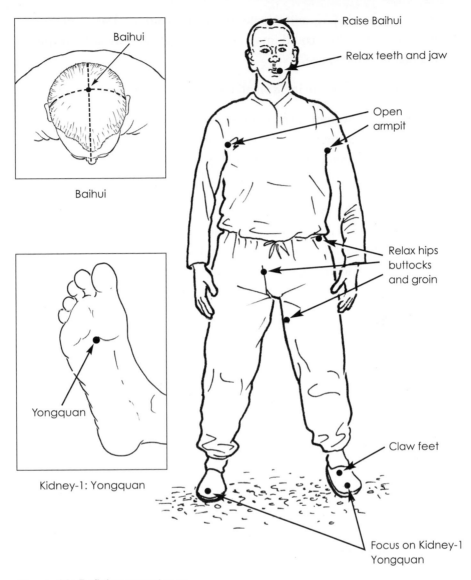

Figure 30: *Refining your stance.*

- Very slightly claw your feet into the ground whenever they are taking your weight. This will activate Kidney-1 (Yongquan) more strongly. However, if this causes tension elsewhere in your body, don't claw your feet until your gain more experience.

- Relax and "soften" your hips, groin, inner thighs, lower back, buttocks, and belly, so that your pelvis feels like it is hanging from the center of your Dantian.

- Relax your teeth, jaw, and shoulders. Then encourage a sense of space in your armpits. You could imagine a small ball of air in each armpit maintaining that space.

- Imagine you are balancing a small book on Baihui (Figure 30).

- Feel your bodyweight relax downward—imagining that it is pooling and therefore filling your legs—rather like sand emptying from the top and filling the bottom half of an egg timer. Thus your legs feel solid and grounded while your torso and head both feel light and buoyant.

- Within your light and buoyant torso, visualize your spinal column as a vertical pillar made of many segments. Imagine those segments drift apart slightly so that air can circulate in those spaces. Do not "will" this to occur, because that will create tension: just gently imagine it. If you can't imagine this or it does not help, just forget about it.

- It can help to imagine you are neck-deep in water (such as a lake) wearing heavy boots that sink into the sediment on the bottom of the "lake." The boots keep your feet totally grounded while your natural buoyancy within the water lengthens your vertebral column and maintains the subtle space under your armpits. All your joints will feel like they are opening, which is good because open joints enable Qi to circulate more freely around your body (Figure 31).

- Your hands should be allowed to concave slightly, which will activate Laogong (Pericardium-8) in the center of your palms. Also, your thumb should be held away from the other fingers so that the web of skin between your thumb and index finger is slightly stretched. This will activate Hegu (Large Intestine-4), Figure 31.

- While standing in this position, it is very useful to make a habit of slowly scanning your body internally from head to feet, noticing any areas of discomfort or areas which just do not feel quite right. Once noticed, do not do anything with these sensations; simply be aware of them. Note that this scanning procedure is a "feeling" exercise and not a visualizing exercise. By feeling, you will eventually acquire the ability to release your internal blockages at will.

- This basic standing position is aimed at awakening your Qi to a certain level prior to continuing with the other Qigong exercises.

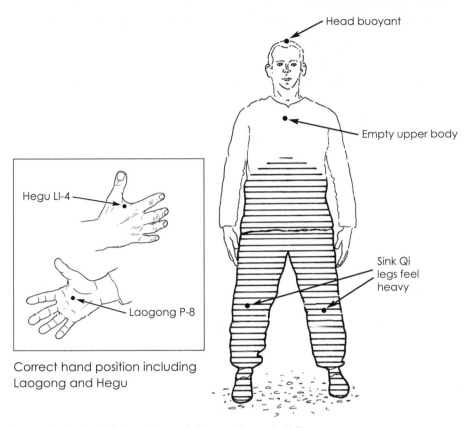

Figure 31: *Top half of body emptying and lower half filling.*

This Qi awakening will take at least ten to thirty minutes to occur, so if you feel it has happened within a minute or two, you have actually stopped well short of the full awakening potential. However, the ability to "feel" internally is cumulative, so don't be discouraged if you do not feel anything during the early days of your practice.

■ Breathing Methods

Within the practice of active Wai Dan (External Elixir) Qigong methods, it is the co-ordination between movement and breath and stillness and breath that unblocks the flow and unlocks the power of Qi within the body.*

The three most familiar methods of breathing in Qigong are natural breathing, normal abdominal breathing, and reverse abdominal breathing.

---

*In most systems of the deeper Nei Dan (Internal Elixir) methods, conscious control of the breath is not practiced. Instead, the Qi is led by the mind alone.

However, if you want to keep the learning process simple, you can focus on learning the Taiji Qigong movements as a sequence before adding any conscious control of the breath. In fact, if you are truly relaxed in your practice, the correct breathing may well occur spontaneously.

Whichever of the three breathing methods you use, inhalation and exhalation should be an unbroken continuum; one leading naturally into the other. When your breathing is especially relaxed, deep and slow, you will experience a pause at the point where inhalation changes to exhalation and exhalation changes to inhalation. However, this should not feel like a break in the continuum, but more like a point of balance as the in-breath naturally transmutes into the out-breath: rather like the stillness of dusk where day meets and yields to night, or dawn where night meets and yields to day.

If you feel your nostrils constrict as you inhale, it's because you are concentrating too hard on breathing rather than allowing it to simply manifest its own strength and pace. Paradoxically, because forcing the breath constricts the nostrils, you get very little extra air for your effort. Good breathing should be without sound and cause little or no sensation or movement within the nostrils.

Natural Breathing

As implied above, it is not a good idea to adapt your breathing in any way until you are well practiced and comfortable with the physical movements of the Qigong. You need to get to the point where the movements flow almost automatically, otherwise you will be splitting your attention between remembering how to breathe and remembering how to move; and messing up both.

Your emotions directly affect your breathing and vice-versa. When you are excited, tense, or angry, you breathe faster and more shallowly, and perhaps irregularly. When you are sad or depressed, you breathe in a sort of collapsed, half-measured way. When you are relaxed and at ease emotionally, you breathe more slowly, deeply, and smoothly.

Therefore, before you begin to practice the Qigong movements, it is important that you are able to calm yourself if excited or motivate yourself if depressed. In other words, you need to regulate your emotions and thoughts.

The key to this is to initially do nothing other than observe your own breathing. The very fact that you are drawing your consciousness inward toward your breathing will begin to "center" your mind. Perhaps not the first time you try it, but with repetition, your mind will habitually become more still as a result. Thus, to encourage good natural breathing, you should:

- Relax.

- Observe and feel your breathing rather than control it.

- Try not to think of anything in the past or future.

- Breathe through your nose.

When you are truly relaxed in natural breathing, you will feel as if your breathing has its own automatic cycle, as if you are passively riding on the rhythm of your breath.

If you get to the point where it feels like the air is breathing you, rather than you breathing the air, then you know you are about as relaxed and centered as it is possible to be.

Getting your breathing sorted (or more accurately, allowing your breathing to return to its natural rhythm) is fundamental to success in Qigong. A good rule to remember is:

> *'Qigong movement should follow the relaxed breath.*
> *The breath should never chase the movement.'*

Adopting this rule will prevent your movements from speeding up, because if you are truly relaxed, your breathing will become slower and deeper, and your movements will follow that pace. Often, when observing some beginners perform Taiji Qigong, it is noticeable that many will increase the pace of the movements as they get bored and try to finish the session more quickly. Consequently their breathing speeds up, which ruins their equanimity. This causes even more impatience to finish as they enter a progressively descending spiral of the breath chasing the movement. As a result, they end up merely going through the motions and completely wasting their time.

Once your breathing and movements are co-ordinated in the natural, relaxed way, you can use your intention, your "Yi," to lead the movements and ultimately lead the Qi. You will feel the Qi as a result of experiencing the movement. Therefore we can expand the rule which states that Qigong movement should follow the breath, to:

> 'The Yi should lead the Qi; the Qi should lead the movement; the movement should follow the breath.'

Normal Abdominal Breathing

Normal abdominal breathing (Zheng Hu Xi) is also called Buddhist breathing. Most young children do this naturally, as do some adults who have remained grounded and centered throughout the stresses of adult life, or have somehow managed to avoid heavy and repetitive stress. However, most adults find they have to re-learn this method of breathing.

When you breathe in, focus on the expansion of your lower belly (Dantian) as your diaphragm naturally descends. In the beginning, you may need to apply conscious effort to your abdominal muscles to make this happen. When you breathe out, relax your abdomen and feel it draw in as your diaphragm ascends. If you can visualize the diaphragm doing this, that's great. If not, just relax the belly as you fix your mind upon your Dantian and it should happen naturally. Encouraging the diaphragm to move more fully in this way will help pump blood around the body and physically massage the organs. Also, because you are focusing on the Dantian, energy will be concentrated there, giving you a grounded center from which vitality will manifest. As you inhale, it will feel like your breath is being pulled all the way down to Dantian, but of course, in reality, the air will go no lower than your diaphragm.

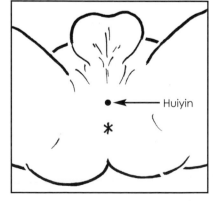

Once you have got your abdominal muscles doing the right thing, you should then incorporate a lift and relaxation of the point known as Huiyin (Ren-1) situated between your anus and genitals (Figure 32). When you contract

Figure 32: *Exact position of Huiyin.*

your belly during exhalation, you should gently pull Huiyin up. When you expand your belly during inhalation, you should gently encourage Huiyin to descend and "open" (Figure 33). In the beginning you may find that you cannot pull up or descend Huiyin. Instead, when you try to do it, you find you pull up or descend your anus. That is normal and still quite effective. After some practice you will begin to feel movement at Huiyin, but accompanied by movement of the anus.

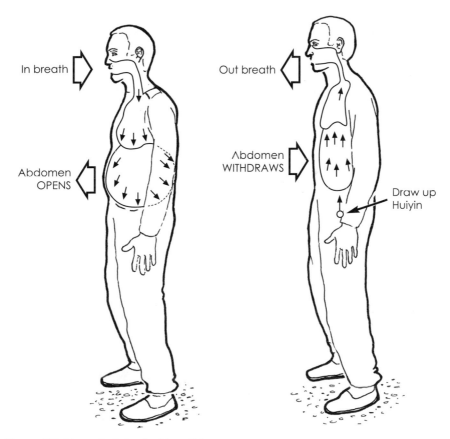

Figure 33: *Normal abdominal breathing.*

As time goes on, you will be able to increase the focus and movement at Huiyin and decrease the movement of the anus. Once you are comfortably established in natural abdominal breathing, you will be able to do it automatically within your Qigong practice while your mind is focused on other specific body parts, sensations, or images.

Reverse Abdominal Breathing

Reverse abdominal breathing (Fan Hu Xi) is also called Daoist breathing, whereby you draw the abdomen in when inhaling and allow the abdomen to relax and expand when exhaling (therefore, the opposite of normal abdominal breathing), Figure 34. The relative pressure difference between the chest cavity and abdominal cavity produces a stronger pumping effect compared to normal abdominal breathing.

Hold up your Huiyin as you inhale and draw your abdomen in. You descend and "open" your Huiyin as you exhale and expand your abdomen. This method is only used for a few breaths at a time, and is used more within Passive Qigongs than Active Qigongs. It is not recommended that you practice this type of breathing unless you have been taught and supervised by an experienced and qualified teacher. If it is practiced incorrectly, it can seriously upset your breathing pattern and distort your Qi flow.

I have described it in this book for the purpose of giving a comprehensive overview of Qigong breathing methods. Therefore, my intention is **NOT** to

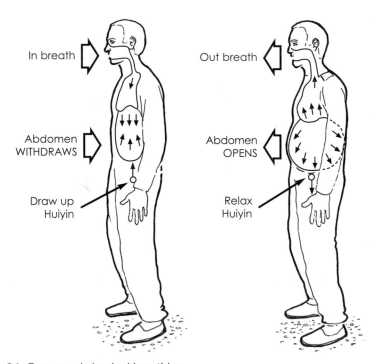

In breath

Abdomen
WITHDRAWS

Draw up
Huiyin

Out breath

Abdomen
OPENS

Relax
Huiyin

Figure 34: *Reverse abdominal breathing.*

encourage you to use the description as an invitation to practice without a teacher. However, for those who are well practiced in this method, reverse breathing can be used effectively and safely within many of the 18 Taiji Qigong exercises.

In all respects, reverse abdominal breathing is more powerful than normal abdominal breathing, but can also cause problems if too much is practiced too soon, or if it is done incorrectly. The biggest pitfall is holding the breath when really the in-breath and out-breath should flow seamlessly from one to the other; at least at the level of Qigong we are describing here.

One reason for doing reverse abdominal breathing rather than normal abdominal breathing is to build up the Defensive Qi (Wei Qi), which circulates predominantly on the exterior of the body. Defensive Qi protects the body from external agents such as excessive heat or cold, or in the context of martial arts training, enables one to more effectively withstand blows from an opponent.

During reverse abdominal breathing, Qi moves more toward the interior of the body with the inhalation and more toward the body's exterior during exhalation. After some practice, this phenomenon can be felt. When you inhale, it will feel as if the Qi is slightly "gripping" your bones. As you exhale, it will feel as if Qi (Defensive Qi) moves toward and even beyond your skin. Practitioners who are accomplished in reverse abdominal breathing find that they can switch from normal to reverse breathing at any time.

Timing the Breath

Your breathing should be in time with your movements, or more accurately, your movements should follow the pace of your relaxed breathing. In general, inhaling accompanies your "opening" movements, and exhaling accompanies your "closing" movements (Figures 35 & 36). Also, you should inhale with rising movements and exhale with sinking movements (Figure 37).**

**In many styles of Taiji Quan, as distinct from Taiji Qigong, the co-ordination of breathing with movement is the opposite, i.e., inhalation takes place as the hands move down or toward the body, and exhalation occurs as the hands move up or away from the body.

In breath

Out breath

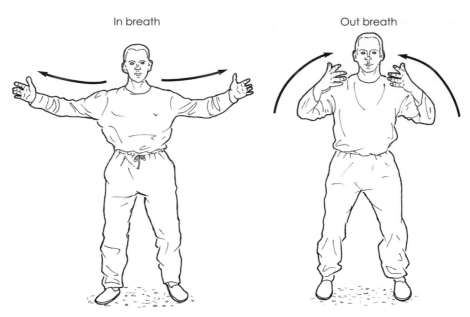

Figure 35: *Breathing pattern for opening and closing movements.*

Out breath

In breath

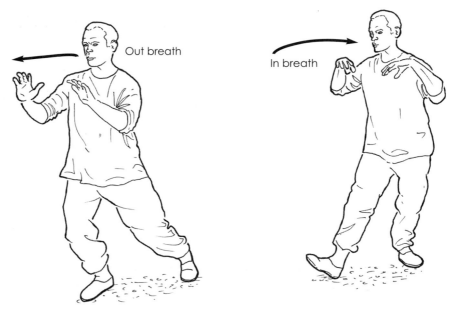

Figure 36: *Breathing pattern for hands going forward and hands withdrawing.*

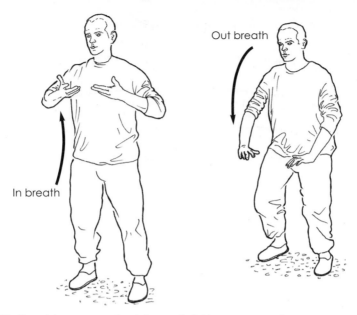

Figure 37: *Breathing pattern for rising and sinking movements.*

Breathing while moving from side to side (Figure 38) can be done one of three ways:

1. Without thinking about the breath.

2. Inhaling when moving to one side, exhaling back to center, and inhaling to the other side.

3. Inhaling as you move to the left and exhaling as you move to the right.

Breathing and moving as one will give you an experience of breathing with your entire body, not just with your lungs. After much practice you will eventually have the sensation that the breath is entering through your skin. Some of it does anyway, but you will begin to appreciate this at an experiential level. At this stage, Qigong will be giving you a real "connection" to your environment. Eventually you may even feel the breath enter through various acupuncture points *(see* page 29), especially if you deliberately focus your mind on those points. As stated earlier, the most important thing to remember about breathing is that the:

> *Movements should follow the breath; the breath should not chase the movements.*

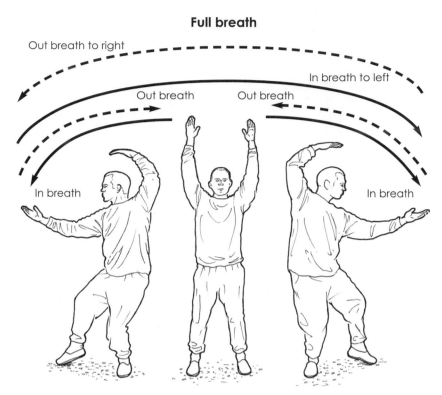

Full breath

Out breath to right

In breath to left

Out breath   Out breath

In breath

In breath

Figure 38: *"Painting the Rainbow" showing inhaling when moving to the side and exhaling back to center, and inhaling to the left and exhaling to the right.*

In other words, only move in time with your relaxed inward and outward breath. Thus, the more relaxed your breathing, the slower your movements will be. Impatience will cause you to rush through the movements to complete them, causing your breathing to speed up. Constantly check yourself for this, because when that happens you are completely wasting your time. You may find it happens when you get to a certain movement. This usually indicates boredom or an energy blockage associated with that movement. Therefore, it is self-diagnostic, giving you an opportunity to reflect upon and address that issue.

Should I Keep My Mouth Open or Closed as I Exhale?

There are different opinions about this, all valid within certain contexts. Most passive Qigongs are practiced with the mouth closed during exhalation, whereas active Qigongs sometimes permit exhalation through the mouth, especially if the movements are big movements, as is the case with many of the Taiji Qigong exercises. However, inhalation is always practiced through the nose, with the mouth closed. Exhalation through the mouth will tend to reduce your Qi slightly, so if you are very debilitated, I would suggest you keep your mouth closed, unless doing so prevents you from exhaling sufficiently. Obviously if your nose is blocked because of a common cold, for example, you will have to open your mouth.

Sometimes, if you are feeling wound up and "full," deliberately exhale through the mouth, with the feeling that the fullness or agitation is dissolving as you do so. Alternatively, breathing out through your nose for two-thirds of your exhalation then out through your mouth for the final third, may suit you.

Whether or not you open or close your mouth, throughout your practice session you should keep the tip of your tongue resting in the center of the roof of your mouth. This makes a connection between the Back Mai and Front Mai, enabling Qi to circulate smoothly around the Small Circulation. There should be no tension in the tongue as you do this, because tension will stagnate the Qi in that area (Figure 39).

Make sure your tongue does not rest against your teeth, because this will break the connection. A positive side-effect of positioning your tongue correctly is that saliva flow is stimulated, which can and should be swallowed to keep your throat moist.

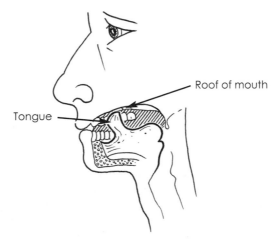

Figure 39: *Correct tongue position on the roof of your mouth.*

Integrating the Vertical and Horizontal "Bows" with the Breath

There is one other consideration to do with breathing, and that is the opening and closing of the Horizontal Arm Bow and the Vertical Spine Bow during reverse abdominal breathing.

The Horizontal Arm Bow is a line connecting the tips of your middle fingers via the posterior surface of your arms and across your upper back. The Vertical Spine Bow is a line from your coccyx, up your spine to the top of your head.

If you stand in the basic Horse Stance (Movement 10) with your arms held relaxed with hands in front of your torso, you will observe that as you breathe in and hold your belly in, your arms will slightly open. This will cause your hands to separate fractionally, and your spine will straighten a little. This is known as "Opening the Bows," (Figure 40).

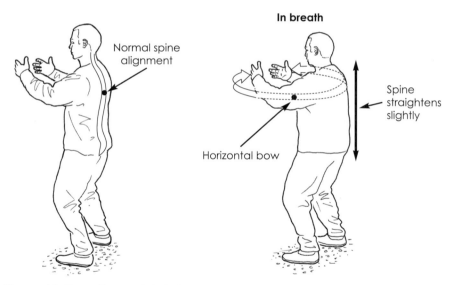

Figure 40: *Open Bow on inhalation.*

As you breathe out and let your belly out, your arms and hands will close a little and your spine will curve very slightly from its slight "S" shape to a slight "C" shape. This is referred to as "Closing the Bows," (Figure 41). You may not notice this so much during the majority of the 18 exercises because the larger movements tend to mask it. However, as time goes on, it will become more apparent. It is well worth just "standing" for several minutes to practice and experience this, which is a Qigong in itself.

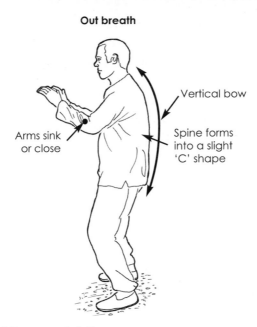

Out breath

Vertical bow

Arms sink
or close

Spine forms
into a slight
'C' shape

Figure 41: *Closed Bow on exhalation.*

Many practitioners do it as a matter of course immediately before and after
their Taiji Qigong session, for up to fifteen minutes at a time. Fifteen to
sixty minutes of just "standing" and observing the bow effect, alongside
focusing on the Small Circulation is a very strong practice. So, if you prefer
not to move, just stand!

■ A Note About Mental Focus

Each exercise has a section called "Mental Focus" within its description,
aimed at maximizing the effect of the exercise. You can practice without
incorporating this and still gain substantial benefits, although less
profoundly. Paradoxically, practicing with the suggested mental focus
will eventually make the exercise easier, because you will be automatically
occupied with that focus, rather than spacing out or getting bored.
The mental focus section is divided into:

• Basic focus.

• Intermediate focus.

• Advanced focus.

Basic Focus

Basic focus usually consists of simply keeping your attention fixed on the Laogong (Pericardium-8) in the center of your palms.

Intermediate Focus

Intermediate focus introduces visualizations to help you connect with the interaction of your Qi with the Qi that surrounds you. In many exercises, the instructions will suggest you extend Qi. This means you should project your mind by visualizing your hands or feet to be moving way beyond their actual physical boundary (Figure 42):

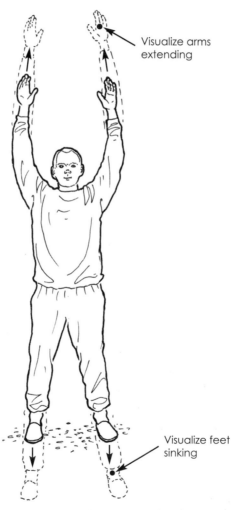

Visualize arms
extending

Visualize feet
sinking

Figure 42: *Qi extended through the fingertips to the sky, and through the feet taking the weight deep into the ground.*

- As your hands move from one side to the other, extend Qi through your fingertips, as if you are painting a rainbow in the sky with your Qi.

- Simultaneously extend Qi into the ground through the foot that is taking most weight, and connect your Qi with Earth Qi.

If you find that there seems too much to visualize at once with any given exercise, focus on just one aspect of the imagery. Extending Qi through your feet will initially be the easiest imagery and give the most powerful feeling. After a while, you will do this automatically, at which point you can incorporate other aspects of the imagery.

Exercises where one foot is placed in front of the other and the weight rocks forward and backward to transfer weight between the feet lend themselves particularly well to a strong feeling of Qi extending into the ground (Figure 43).

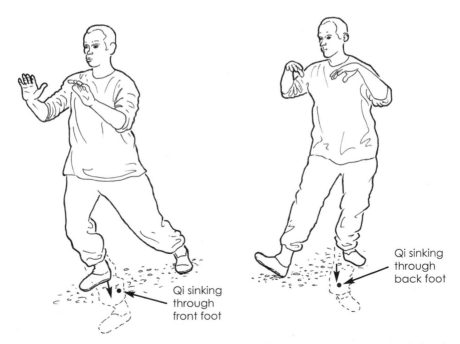

Qi sinking through front foot

Qi sinking through back foot

Figure 43: *"Pushing Waves," showing Qi extended through the feet as each foot in turn takes the weight.*

Note that the terms "visualize" and "imagery" refer to clues as to what you may eventually feel. Most people have better powers of visual imagery compared to their ability to feel or sense Qi. Once you can really feel what you are visualizing, you will at that stage have developed your Wai Dan Qigong to quite a high level.

Advanced Focus

Advanced focus incorporates the Small Circulation of Qi (see page 43) as an alternative to the prescribed intermediate visualizations. This works particularly well during exercises that consist largely of movements in the vertical plane rather than twisting or sideways movements. For example, exercises 1, 2, 4, 6, 11, 12, 13, 15, 17, and 18. The best method for doing this in the context of Taiji Qigong is to use what is known as the single breath reverse breathing cycle (see page 62 and Figure 44).

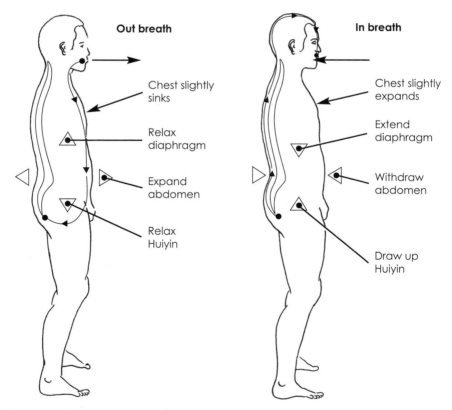

Figure 44: *Single breath reverse breathing cycle.*

- As you exhale, draw your attention from your nose, down the midline of your body to the tailbone.

- As you inhale, draw your attention from the tailbone to the nose—continuing with another circuit during the next breath and so on.

However, I reiterate once more: **Do not practice reverse breathing unless you have been tutored and supervised by an experienced teacher**. If you are an impatient person who believes that advanced practices can be quickly mastered from simply reading a book, please be careful and reflect upon the reasons for your impatience. Forgetting about the breathing altogether is also a valid approach at this level, for you are likely to be breathing appropriately without having to think about it.

■ A Note About Internal Effects

Some of the exercises also have a section called "Internal Effects." After a period of dedicated regular practice, the effects described will begin to occur. These effects are in addition to the natural increase of Qi circulating smoothly throughout the channels and within the Small Circulation. In other words, enhancing the free flow of Qi throughout the body is an internal effect common to all of the exercises to a greater or lesser extent, so the other effects listed are additional effects.

IMPORTANT! You will notice that in Exercise 1, the knees are bending when the arms are raised (Figure 45). This is because in the beginning we want to establish a clear awareness of Heaven Qi moving through our body from above to below. Qi moving predominantly in this direction, rather than upward through the body, is necessary for general wellbeing. In other words, we need to establish a strong sense of "grounding" before we proceed further.

So, whenever you raise your arms without raising your center of gravity, the Qi deep within your body will sink more noticeably downward toward your feet, into the ground. Practice Exercise 1, and experience this for yourself. To exaggerate this effect, try raising your hands quickly. You should feel a sudden heaviness in your buttocks and feet as you do so.

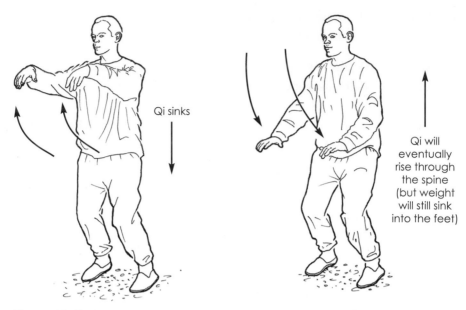

Qi sinks

Qi will eventually rise through the spine (but weight will still sink into the feet)

Figure 45: *Beginning Movement: Qi sinks into the legs as the arms are raised and lowered.*

When you lower your arms, you will still experience weight sinking into your feet, but after a lot of practice, you should begin to simultaneously experience your spine "opening" and Qi rising upward through your spine.

After even more practice, you should eventually experience a general spreading and expansion of Qi in all directions. This will result in a feeling of being well-grounded but light and buoyant.

Note that this exercise is very commonly taught another way; i.e., the legs bend when the arms are lowered and straighten when the arms are raised. This is equally valid. As previously mentioned, there are many versions of this Qigong taught.

You will notice that in Exercise 2, the legs bend when the arms are lowered and straighten when the arms are raised (Figure 46). This is designed to encourage a raising of Earth Qi into the body, to complement the descent of Heaven Qi into the body. This must be done without losing your sense of being grounded. Experiential feelings such as this are difficult to convey in words. Experiment and play with these exercises a little to discover the nuances for yourself.

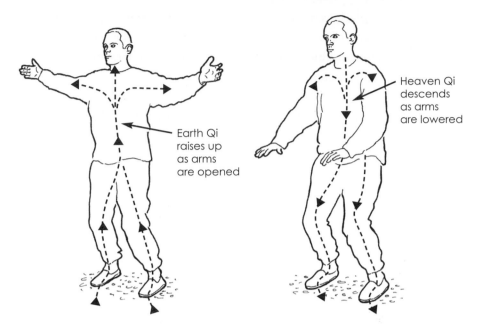

Figure 46: *Opening the Chest: Earth Qi raises through the legs as the arms are raised. When the arms are lowered, Heaven Qi descends through the body from above.*

For those exercises which are predominantly in the vertical plane (namely, 1, 2, 4, 6, 11, 12, 13, 15, 17, and 18), rather than those which largely involve twisting or sideways movements, the following internal effects will occur to some extent, depending on your level of practice and the natural "openness" of your Qi reservoirs. This is particularly so if the single breath reverse breathing cycle is used as the mental focus.

As your Qi descends through your feet into the ground, Earth Qi will enter your body through K-1 (Yongquan) and to some extent, Ren-1 (Huiyin). This does not mean that you are pulling Earth Qi up. It means that your Human Qi (your sense of weight, and your mind) descends into the earth and absorbs Earth Qi, rather like blotting paper absorbs ink. This Qi will then enter the Back Mai that runs up the back of your spine and head, to supplement the Qi flowing within the Small Circulation. Some Qi may also move up the Middle Mai from the Lower Dantian, depending on the level of Qi in Dantian and the "openness" of the Middle Mai.

If you are particularly centered and well practiced, as you lower your arms, Heaven Qi will enter Du-20 (Baihui) and descend down the Front Mai situated along the midline of your torso, to further supplement Qi flowing through the Small Circulation.

Meanwhile, an increased flow of Qi will emanate from Ren-17 (Shanzhong) on your breastbone, and move along your Pericardium channel, charging Pericardium-8 (Laogong) with Qi.

Also, as your arms descend during exhalation, any physical, mental, and emotional tension will unblock and dissolve, thus transforming itself into free-flowing Qi. Within the relevant exercises, this description of effects will be abridged to simply read:

'Heaven Qi and Earth Qi may naturally supplement your Small Circulation. Any emotional and physical tensions will transform into free-flowing Qi.'

■ A Note About Benefits

The benefits described with each exercise are explained using the concepts of traditional Chinese medicine theory, which like Qigong, are firmly rooted in the principles of Daoism. Indeed, Qigong is generally seen as an aspect of Chinese medicine, either as a primary healing system through the practice of medical Qigong, or as an adjunct to improve one's health.

Hopefully, I have described these effects in a clear, concise way that makes some sense. However, traditional Chinese medicine differs in many ways to Western medical theory. For example, the word Liver in the Chinese context covers a whole spectrum of body and mind interrelationships and connections, far beyond the liver's physiology as described in Western medicine. Hence, when referring to an organ or concept in the traditional Chinese sense, it is the accepted custom to begin the relevant word with a capital letter. For example, "Liver" refers to the Chinese medicine concept of Liver, whereas "liver" refers to the anatomical liver organ in Western medicine.

A benefit common to all 18 exercises within Taiji Qigong is the strengthening of what can be called the "Earth Element" within us.

Having discussed Earth Qi (*see* pages 10–11), we can consider the Earth Element to be the qualities of Earth Qi we hold within ourselves. These qualities can all be summed up as aspects of support. The concept of support in relation to the earth becomes clear when we consider how the earth literally supports us by providing the ground upon which we stand, our shelter, and the food we eat. It is the center of our existence in every way.

When the qualities of planet earth are strong within us; in other words, when we have a strong Earth Element, we exhibit the following qualities.

We have a strong feeling of being supported and of being able to support others. In a woman, a literal example of this is being able to provide milk for her newborn baby. To the baby she is the center, providing care and nourishment on all levels. Therefore, if our Earth Element is weak, we might feel like nobody is supporting our needs and are therefore too insecure to truly support others.

Strong Earth Qi within us will also enable us to assimilate the essence of the earth, which to us is food. Hence, a robust digestive system indicates that our Earth Qi is strong. If our Earth Element is weak, we can develop digestive problems and under-nourishment based on the inability to assimilate enough essential nutrients.

For us, the gravity and solidity of planet earth holds everything together. Hence, our ability to physically hold ourselves together is manifested by the tone of our flesh and the fact that our connective tissues support our vital organs. If our Earth Element is weak, the tone of our muscles and connective tissues may weaken, causing a general sagging of the body, which at worst may lead to such things as varicose veins or the prolapse of certain organs.

It is because we have the ground to stand upon that we have a familiar base or point of reference from which to look up at the heavens. The solidity of the earth enables us to recognize the comparative "emptiness" of the sky; and so a solid feeling of being grounded enables us to open up to the vibrations of the "heavens."

This means that because Earth Qi enters us, mostly through our feet, we are able to open up to Heaven Qi, which enters mostly through our head. This is similar to a plant rooting itself into the ground so that it can reach up to the sunlight, which is the plant's most important form of Heaven Qi. If the Earth Element within us is weak, we could have trouble with physical balance, much like a plant with shallow roots. Also, the lack of a stable base will prevent us from having the polarity to connect with the more subtle aspects of Heaven Qi, such as intuition.

In practice, this means that by being more grounded within our stances, we will naturally allow a greater downward movement of Heaven Qi through our bodies. This is important to understand, because a fundamental principle of Qigong is that the unimpeded flow of Heaven Qi moving down and through us from above is a key factor in maintaining both physical health and emotional stability.

Being grounded in reality; or to use a very apt expression, 'having our feet firmly on the ground', gives us a stable base from which to perceive things clearly. This is in contrast to those who are not grounded, who are often referred to as "spaced out." Thus, the ability to perceive and think clearly is largely dependent upon being well connected to Earth Qi, which in turn anchors our mind and enables us to use our thinking abilities (our Yi, which can then lead our Qi!). Consequently, if our Earth Element is weak, our thinking process will be confused rather than lucid. For one thing, this will make the imagery practice within Qigong difficult.

In brief, most standing or moving Qigong exercises such as Taiji Qigong, by virtue of the great emphasis placed upon having a firmly rooted stance, draw abundant Earth Qi into our body, which strengthens our Earth Element. The polarity caused by being "earthed" through the feet creates sufficient polarity between Yin (earth) and Yang (sky/space) to attract Heaven Qi through the head (although both Earth Qi and Heaven Qi are also slightly absorbed through other parts of the body). The benefits of this are: better digestion, clearer thinking, better visceral and muscular tone, stronger polarity between Heaven Qi and Earth Qi causing greater uptake of these energies, a deeper sense of feeling supported and a greater capacity to give support to others.

The other universal benefit of all Taiji Qigong exercises is a smoother flow and distribution of Qi and blood. This is because the movements of the exercises have a fluid, wave-like quality that gently stimulates the circulation of blood, particularly through the joints, thus helping to lubricate them. This helps to inhibit osteoarthritic degeneration within joints, because such fluid-like movements encourage the smooth flow of Qi and a more even distribution of blood, particularly to the joints, which according to Chinese medicine are functions largely controlled by the Liver. All the exercises therefore promote these Liver functions, ensuring that blood reaches and nourishes the joints and the "sinews" (tendons, muscles, and ligaments), as well as ironing out the kinks within our Qi which can block or disturb its flow though the various channels. A smoother flow of Qi also impacts on our mind, causing a greater emotional equanimity.

If you add all those things together by getting it right, you should feel pretty good! However, absorb the meaning of this little maxim: 'Reading about it might make you do it, but doing it makes it happen!'

As a bonus for anyone involved in Qi-based bodywork, such as shiatsu or tuina, the increase in Qi level in general—plus the particular increase in Qi reaching the hands—will make your treatments much more powerful.

■ A Note About Motivation

Sometimes you will not want to do these Qigong exercises; or you will start off, but be totally uninspired to continue. For some people this happens very occasionally, while for others it happens most of the time. You will probably fall somewhere in between. Usually it goes in phases, so you might go for periods of time where you can't wait to start and don't want to stop. Other phases will include periods of total ambivalence or inertia. This is quite normal, and it helps to know that you're not the only one.

Sometimes, when the will to finish your sessions (or even start them) is weak, it can be helpful to play suitably evocative music as you practice. Choose something that has the correct rhythm and creates the right atmosphere for you. Music can be very powerful, with the ability to transform a mood very quickly. The right music may also help you to concentrate better. Use it as a tool, but don't allow it to become indispensable within your Qigong, otherwise you might find it difficult to practice spontaneously; for example, while out on a walk in the countryside.

■ Possible Side-Effects

The benefits of doing Qigong are overwhelmingly positive. You will have more energy, better concentration, increased equanimity of mind and emotional stability, improved posture and flexibility, greater endurance, better digestion, greater body awareness, greater appreciation of your personal space and of your surroundings, more awareness of other people's space, and an intuitive insight into other people's level and distribution of Qi.

However, you may or may not experience some mild reactions from time to time, but these are also ultimately positive as they either reflect some sort of cleansing reaction, or they indicate a problem with your practice that you can then correct. Those reactions which are physical sensations usually happen as you are practicing or shortly after. However, you are unlikely to experience these reactions to any degree unless you are doing a lot of focused and intense Qigong. Some of the symptoms listed, such as flatulence or diarrhoea may of course occur for other reasons, unrelated to your Qigong.

The most common side-effects are itching and pain in various parts of the body. This can indicate an area of your body where the Qi is unable to get through, thus causing an accumulation or "fulness" in that area. This is very useful, as it highlights a specific area to focus on. It is very commonly felt in the shoulders, back, neck, and arms. The solution is to "open" the joints of the fingers, hand, wrist, elbow, and shoulder.

Itching or pain can also reflect a stagnation of Qi in that area; in which case it needs to be encouraged to dissolve or transmuted through continual refinement of your practice. These sensations may then simply disappear as your Qi begins to circulate more smoothly.

Another result of a chronic Qi blockage may be a build up of poisons. As the Qi and blood is circulated more effectively, these substances will be brought to the liver for detoxification.

Other possible side-effects are listed, illustrating the reaction and the reason for the reaction.

Burping and Flatulence

As your Qi starts to move and strengthen in your Lower Dantian, stagnant gases will be dislodged and flushed out.

Bloating of Intestines

Often this is caused by closing rather than opening the lumbar vertebrae, possibly through holding and developing a hollow back. The resultant constriction of the nerves emanating from the lumbar spine will interrupt the natural movement of the intestines, causing a backlog of gas.

Tingling, Swelling, Pain, or Hot Clammy Sensations in the Hands, and Less Commonly, the Feet

Stagnant Qi most readily accumulates in the hands, feet, and bowels, if it is not transformed. Massaging yourself between your fingers after exercises will help disperse the stagnation.

Sensation of a Cold Wind Leaving the Hands

A less common phenomenon, indicating a significant discharge of Qi that could not be transformed.

Diarrhoea

This can be a natural cleansing reaction as your body strengthens and re-balances itself through Qigong. It is most likely to happen for a short time when your lumbar vertebrae start to "open up."

Excessive Salivation

This is the normal response to holding the tip of your tongue on the roof of your mouth. It serves to lubricate the throat. If excessive, move your tongue forward slightly, but not so far as to touch your teeth.

Spontaneous Movement

You are very unlikely to experience this within Taiji Qigong, but if you do it will be during the still phases, most likely during Exercise 18. It will only happen if your mind is relaxed, "empty," and dwelling in the present. Hence, it is a good sign. True spontaneous movement will be experienced as originating from your Lower Dantian. However, if it does not stop, or occurs at other times (both extremely unlikely), seek out an experienced Qigong instructor for advice.

Cold Sensation in Head

This indicates poor circulation at a deep level, which suggests you should practice a Wai Dan Qigong such as Taiji Qigong as regularly as possible.

Sensation of Cold Coming Out from the Base of Your Neck (at First Thoracic Vertebra)

This can reflect weak Kidneys and lack of Qi/Heat in the Gate of Vitality usually reflected in weak sexual energy. Again, Qigong highlighted the problem, yet Qigong can be a big part of the solution.

Blistering and Burning of the Palms Shortly after You Begin Your Qigong Exercises

Very unusual, but can happen if certain "centers" or "pathways" are opened prematurely or incorrectly by "transmission" or "invocation" within some energy-based healing disciplines. If it happens to you, go back to the person who "opened you up" and ask them to "close you down."

■ The Concept of Distorted Qi

In Qigong, there are two ways of conceptualizing the nature of discomfort and the resolution of it. One idea is that all forms of discomfort, whether physical or emotional, ultimately represent distorted Qi, which must be dissolved or transformed into free-flowing Qi before the discomfort will subside. Another view is that this distorted Qi is better expelled than transformed. Within the latter view, this distorted Qi is referred to as either "negative" or "sick" Qi. In reality, it is likely that elements of both views hold true.

Distorted Qi can also refer to negative attitudes of mind, especially repressed or stuck emotions. For example, if you hold the image of flushing out or "letting go of" stored anger or envy during a Qigong exercise, you are in a way, expelling negative Qi. By contrast, the "transforming" viewpoint prefers the image of allowing the emotion to dissolve or transform simply by being mindfully aware of its existence.

The enhanced Qi circulation acquired through Qigong exercises will naturally transform this blocked energy (which is what all pain and repressed or stuck emotions represent) into free-flowing energy.

Actually, within the "transforming" viewpoint there are two methods for resolving stuck emotions. One way is as just described, i.e., that recognizing the problem will unlock it, enabling the Qigong to transform and move it. The other approach is that an unwanted emotional state is best transformed during Qigong exercises by supplanting it with the opposite feeling or attitude.

For example, if you feel angry, imagine that you are surrounded by a halo of joy. However, if you are really stuck emotionally, it is extremely difficult to realistically reproduce another emotion, otherwise you wouldn't be stuck. On balance, allowing emotions to dissolve through mindfulness is used more than supplanting one emotion for another.

Of course, problems in the body can initiate negative mental attitudes; for example, constant pain or fatigue can lead to frustration and despair. Similarly, repressed emotions can lead to physical problems; for example, constant worry leading to a stomach ulcer. Hence, there is not always a clear distinction between mentally generated Qi distortions and physically generated Qi distortions. A major characteristic of Daoism—and therefore Qigong and Chinese medicine—is that it recognizes and explores the integration of the physical, mental, and emotional.

To express the transformation or expulsion of distorted Qi with a simple summary, we can say that distorted Qi is either transformed or driven out by the robust circulation of Original Qi as it flows through the channels (Jing Luo) and reservoirs of Qi (Jing Mai). Pain or illness is a reflection of the Original Qi not circulating, for whatever reason, with sufficient strength to transform or expel the disturbed Qi. Health therefore depends on the robust and smooth flow of Original Qi.

PART III

The 18 Movements of Taiji Qigong

■ Notes to Help Your Practice

1. Unless otherwise stated within the instructions for any of the exercises described, the breathing should be natural. If you are proficient in normal (Buddhist) breathing, you can use that method if preferred. Reverse (Daoist) breathing can also be used if you have been taught this by an experienced teacher and you are confident you can do it correctly. Even then, don't overdo it. Whichever method of breathing you choose, the following pattern will apply:

    *   Breathe in through the nose and out through the nose, or out through the mouth if preferred; but keep the tip of your tongue touching the roof of your mouth all the time.

    *   Breathe in with opening and/or rising movements; breathe out with closing and/or descending movements.

    *   Breathe in as you move to the left and out as you move to the right; or if preferred, breathe in as you move sideways (left or right) away from the center line and out as you move back to the center line.

If you are having trouble with your co-ordination while learning the form, forget about your breathing until you can remember the movements (*see* Figures 39–41).

2. A shortened name is given for each exercise, often prefixed or suffixed by the remainder of the full title in brackets. Alternative names are also given where applicable.

3. Bending the legs refers to an angle of 30–40 degrees. Straightening the legs means legs straight but without bracing the knees. The knees should therefore be "soft." Straighten or outstretch the arms means arms straight but with elbows unlocked. Basically, there are few if any moving Qigong exercises where the elbows or knees lock out straight, because to do so would block the flow of Qi through those joints.

4. Wherever Dantian is written, it refers to the Lower Dantian, unless otherwise specified.

■ "Raising the Heels" Variation

For the advanced practitioner, the exercises where you raise your arms on inhalation and sink down on exhalation, i.e., those done in a vertical plane rather than twisting or side bending, lend themselves to the single breath reverse breathing cycle. Such exercises can also lend themselves to a variation whereby you raise both heels off the ground as you inhale, and then sink your heels back to the ground as you exhale.

Many practitioners like to add the heel raising option occasionally, just for a change (Figure 47). However, it is very difficult to maintain a sense of your Qi descending down and out through your feet if you raise your heels. That's not surprising, since its purpose is to help develop a feeling of internal lifting of the pelvic floor associated with the raising of Ren-1 (Huiyin) during reverse abdominal breathing. As such, I would recommend you avoid this heel raising variant unless or until you have fully mastered grounding your Qi throughout each exercise.

When raising the heels, you will naturally contract your calf muscles. This has the added bonus of helping to regulate your adrenal hormones through a reflex connecting the calf muscles to the adrenal glands. Raising the heels is also good for developing balance.

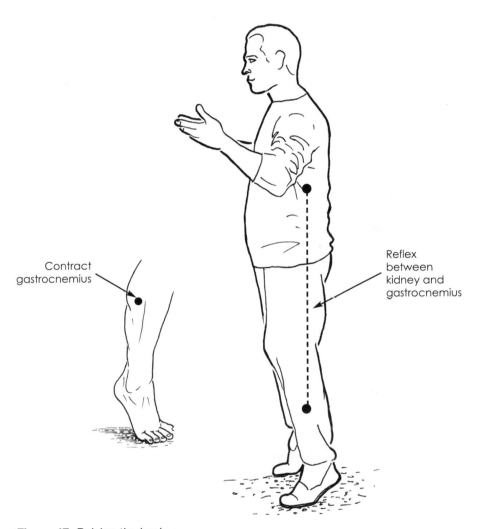

Contract
gastrocnemius

Reflex
between
kidney and
gastrocnemius

Figure 47: *Raising the heels.*

1

Beginning (...Movement)

■ Stance and Movements

Stand naturally with your arms relaxed by your side, feet parallel about shoulder-width apart and your knees very slightly bent.

Look directly ahead or very slightly down, with eyelids open, but relaxed. (Allow your eyes to close if facing directly into the rising or setting sun.)

Your back should be straight but relaxed throughout. Your elbows should be unlocked and your relaxed fingers will naturally curl slightly.

As you inhale

* Raise your arms forward with palms down, to slightly higher than shoulder height. Bend your knees slightly as you do this (page 73 under **IMPORTANT!** within Internal Effects). Ensure your knees do not project beyond your toes.

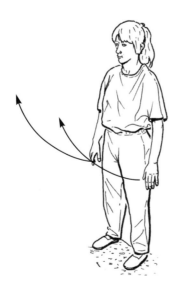
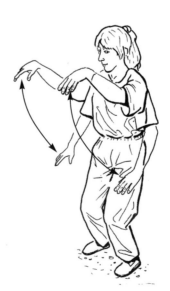

As you exhale

- Allow your hands to gradually sink down to waist height; slightly straightening your knees as you do so.

■ Mental Focus

- If you find it difficult to keep your neck relaxed and upright, visualize something light in weight balancing on your head throughout the movement. Before you begin to move, fix your mind on Dantian for 2–3 breaths.

Basic Focus

- Focus your attention on Laogong (Pericardium-8).

- Use natural breathing (page 58).

Intermediate Focus
Option 1

- As you lower your arms, extend Qi from Yongquan (Kidney-1) far into the ground, so you feel you are connecting with Earth Qi at a deep level.

- Then, when you raise your arms, feel that your Qi descends from your Lower Dantian into the ground to meet with and absorb Earth Qi. As such, you should adopt natural breathing, or use normal breathing so that Ren-1 (Huiyin) opens as your arms are raised during inhalation.

Option 2
If you are feeling "full" and "blocked" and want to dissolve or transform this fullness or blockage of Qi:

- As you raise your arms and inhale, imagine clear water (if you feel hot) or warm fine sand (if you feel cold) is being sucked up through Yongquan (Kidney-1) into your legs and filling your entire body, absorbing and transforming the tensions, stress, pain, anger, etc.

- As you lower your arms and exhale, feel the water or sand flood out through the soles of your feet and deep into the earth, to be replaced with fresh water or sand during your next inhalation.

- Use natural or normal breathing, although you can also use reverse breathing if proficient.

Option 3

If you are feeling "empty" and listless and want to absorb fresh Qi:

- Imagine you are enveloped within a ball of pure white light or fluid-like nectar which you absorb as you do the movements.

Advanced Focus

- Use the single breath reverse breathing cycle (page 62), or natural breathing (page 58).

- Occasionally, it is useful to use the heel raising option to facilitate this focus, i.e., raise your heels as you inhale and gently sink your heels back down as you exhale.

■ Internal Effects

If your focus is on the single breath reverse breathing cycle, Earth Qi will enter through your feet and sometimes through Ren-1 (Huiyin) into the Small Circulation. Heaven Qi might also enter the Small Circulation via Du-20 (Baihui). In addition, Qi will flow from Ren-17 (Shanzhong) along your Pericardium channel, charging your palms (Laogong) with Qi.

This effect in other exercises will be abridged to read: "Heaven Qi and Earth Qi may naturally supplement your Small Circulation. Any emotional and physical tensions will transform into free flowing Qi" (see A Note About Internal Effects, page 73).

■ Benefits

As with all these exercises, this one has all the benefits listed under A Note about Benefits, page 76, plus:

Calms the mind, because …

- Absorbing the cool Yin quality of Earth Qi during the rising movement and dissolving or transforming mental and physical tensions during the descending movement will sedate the Liver Qi if it is overactive. Overactive Liver Qi has an agitated quality and can rise up to the head, causing you to lose your composure. Blocked Liver Qi can create anger and frustration, which is the antithesis of calmness.

2

Opening the Chest

■ Stance and Movements

On a Single Slow In-Breath

- Raise your arms with palms down as you did in the previous exercise, but only to chest height. Slightly straighten or bend your knees according to your level of experience (page 73, under **IMPORTANT!** within Internal Effects).

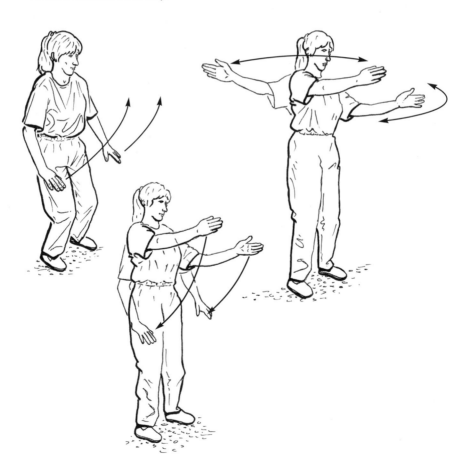

- Without pausing, turn your palms to face your chest with fingertips turned toward each other.

- Open your arms out to the sides.

On a Single Slow Exhalation

- Bring your arms and palms back together until they are shoulder-width apart.

- Then turn them downward and lower them to waist height.

Note

- Don't open your arms so much that your neck and upper back tighten up, because you should maintain "openness" between your shoulder blades.

- Elbows should remain slightly bent.

■ Mental Focus

Basic Focus

- Focus your attention on Laogong (Pericardium-8).

- Use natural breathing (page 58).

Intermediate Focus
Options 1 and 2

- Focus is the same as for Exercise 1.

Advanced Focus
Option 1

- Use the single breath reverse breathing cycle (page 72).

Option 2

- Using normal or reverse abdominal breathing as you raise your arms to chest height, be open to the possibility of sensing a sky-blue light traveling from your Lower Dantian up the Middle Mai to your Middle Dantian.

- When you turn your palms toward your chest, feel that Laogong in the center of your palms connects with the Qi you have just raised to the chest.

- As you spread your arms sideways, feel Laogong pulling Qi out of Shanzhong (Ren-17), to spiral open into a large bubble of Qi in front of your chest. If you feel like distributing some positive Qi in the form of compassion or goodwill toward others, let the Qi bubble disperse and radiate to all beings. If you have some anger, grief, or other such emotions, you can hold the idea that those emotions are within your Qi bubble, to be transformed by the neutrality of a surrounding Universal Qi.

- Gather in your Qi bubble (imbued with fresh Qi) when closing your arms and press it toward the floor as your hands descend, so that you have a large ball of Qi reaching from the floor to your Lower Dantian.

- As you inhale and raise your arms again, feel that the Qi is pulled into the Middle Mai via the Lower Dantian and raised up as before. In addition, you may like to add to that Qi by drawing in fresh Earth Qi through the soles of your feet.

■ Internal Effects

The effects are the same as described for Exercise 1: Heaven Qi and Earth Qi may naturally supplement your Small Circulation. Any emotional and physical tensions will transform into free-flowing Qi.

■ Benefits

Opens and expands Qi in the chest, thereby strengthening the heart and lungs which helps **reduce depression, because ...**

- The Heart affects, and is most affected by, joy/excitement.

- The Lung affects, and is most affected by, grief/depression.

3

Painting a Rainbow (sometimes called "Dancing With the Rainbow")

■ Stance and Movements

Raise your hands above your head, palms facing each other. Hold them slightly wider than shoulder-width apart, with elbows relaxed.

Option 1
As you inhale

- Lean your hands to the left as you bend your right knee and move your pelvis to the right; thus forming a crescent shape with your body, and simultaneously swivel your left toes to face the left.

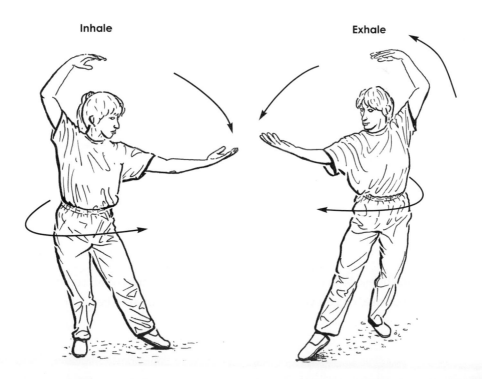

Inhale   Exhale

As you exhale

- Lean your hands to the right as you bend your left knee and move your pelvis to the left, and simultaneously swivel your right toes to face the right.

Option 2
As you inhale

- Same as Option 1: Lean your hands to the left as you bend your right knee and move your pelvis to the right; thus forming a crescent shape with your body, and simultaneously swivel your left toes to face the left.

As you exhale

- Look at your upturned left palm. Meanwhile your right palm is held above your head projecting Qi from P-8 (Laogong) into Du-20 (Baihui).

As you inhale

- Bring your hands all the way to the right, pelvis to the left, etc.

As you exhale

- Look at your right hand. This time your left palm will project Qi from P-8 into Du-20 (*see* Figure 38, page 66, which illustrates the co-ordination of breath with the movement).

Note

- When you swivel your foot, you may wish to hold the heel of that foot off the ground. Doing so or not doing so are both acceptable and common practices.

- At no time during a single repetition of the movement should either hand drop below shoulder height.

- You can choose to keep your hands up for the duration of all repetitions of the exercise, or you can bring them down to your side between repetitions.

■ Mental Focus

Basic Focus

- Focus your attention on Laogong (Pericardium-8).

- Use natural breathing (page 58).

Intermediate Focus
Option 1

- If your head is feeling hot and/or you have a headache, feel that you are pouring cool water from Laogong into the top of your head, through Baihui.

- If your head is feeling full, as if it wants to burst, imagine that you are pulling strands of Qi out of your head with the palms of your hands.

Option 2

- As your hands move from one side to the other, extend Qi through your fingertips, as if you are painting a rainbow with your Qi high in the sky.

- Simultaneously extend Qi into the ground through the foot that is taking most weight, and connect your Qi with Earth Qi.

Note

- If you find it difficult to focus on all these things at once, choose to focus on extending Qi through the feet **OR** through the hands. You could change the focus to the other option at intervals through the exercise.

■ Internal Effects

The raising up, holding and lowering of the arms, coupled with the side to side movements regulate the Qi in the Triple Heater channel (Figure 11, page 23). If you do not lower your arms, the effect is more directed to increasing Qi in the Heart channel (Figure 6, page 22).

■ Benefits

Strengthens the stomach and digestion because ...

- All Qigong exercises that shift weight from one leg to the other create a strong connection with Earth Qi through the weight bearing foot (page 74). Particularly with this exercise, the fact that your arms are held in a raised position will encourage the Earth Qi to be absorbed upward beyond the Lower Dantian into the stomach organ.

Strengthens the heart because ...

- The position of your arms held above shoulder level throughout this exercise will cause Qi to fill your Heart and Pericardium channels. These run along the front (medial and anterior) surface of your arms, from your chest to your hands (Figure 6, page 22 and Figure 10, page 23).

Strengthens your resistance to disease because ...

- The Triple Heater supplies and regulates Qi flow directly to the internal organs, ensuring their efficient functioning. As such, it harmonizes the functions of respiration, digestion, and elimination.

May reduce headaches because ...

- Laogong point in the center of the palm is connecting and transmitting Qi as a calming, cooling influence to the Baihui point on the top of the head. However, don't do this exercise if you feel you have hot or cold clammy palms or a cold wind-like feeling coming from your hands, because this means you have a significant Qi distortion that is moving through your hands, as yet un-dissolved or un-transformed. If that is the case, repeat Exercise 1 as a substitute for this exercise.

4

Separating the Clouds

■ Stance and Movements

From the previous exercise, your hands descend sideways with palms turned outward, as you bend your knees and exhale. Your wrists cross in front of your lower belly, palms turned toward you.

As you inhale

- Continue crossing your arms in front of you, raising them overhead.

- Straighten your knees as you do so.

As you exhale

- Your arms descend again and continue the desired number of repetitions as a continuous circular motion.

- To conclude, hold your hands in front of your Dantian, one hand overlapping the other.

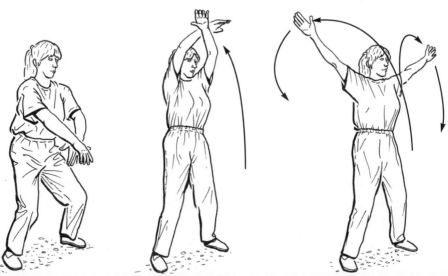

■ Mental Focus

Basic Focus

- Focus your attention on Laogong (Pericardium-8).

- Use natural breathing (page 58).

Intermediate Focus
Option 1

- Feel that you are gathering fresh Earth Qi through your feet as you sink your feet into the ground during inhalation. This supportive Earth Qi fills your body, absorbing or transforming any feelings of depression or of being unsupported.

- As you exhale, Heaven Qi is attracted into your body through the top of your head.

Option 2

- If you feel strong and disposed toward helping others, feel that you are absorbing the supportive, nurturing strength of Earth Qi through the soles of your feet as you inhale. You can then radiate that strength out of Laogong in your palms to all beings around you, near and far, as you exhale.

Advanced Focus

- As you raise your arms above your head with reverse breathing, visualize a sky-blue light ascend the Middle Mai to the top of your head.

- As you lower your arms, feel Qi descend from the top of your head down the Front Mai into the Lower Dantian.

- With each subsequent repetition of the exercise, either follow the single breath reverse breathing cycle (page 72), or modify it so that the Qi is visualized as ascending the Middle Mai rather than the Back Mai.

■ Internal Effects

The absorbed Heaven Qi and Earth Qi may naturally supplement your Small Circulation. Any Qi distortions are encouraged to dissolve or transform (*see* A Note About Internal Effects, page 73). With the advanced focus described above, this exercise particularly moves Qi through the Middle Mai and descends Qi down the Front Mai into the Lower Dantian.

■ Benefits

Benefits the heart and lungs because ...

- The movement of the arms during this exercise flushes Qi along all the channels in the arm, but particularly along the Lung, Heart, and Pericardium channels in the chest.

Clears the head, awakening the brain because ...

- The stimulation of the lungs and heart increase the oxygen uptake of the blood, which is also more efficiently pumped up to the head because of the large upward movement of the arms.

5

Arm Rolling (...in Fixed Stance)
(sometimes called "Back Swinging Monkey")

■ Stance and Movements

Stay in the basic stance and raise your arms outstretched in front of your chest. The left palm faces downward a few inches over the right palm that faces upward; so that P-8 (Laogong) in both palms face each other and "connect."

As you inhale

- Descend your hand past your thigh and behind you, in an arc, so that it ends up at shoulder height. Keep your eyes fixed on that hand all the way.

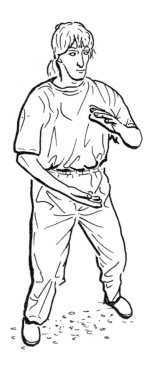
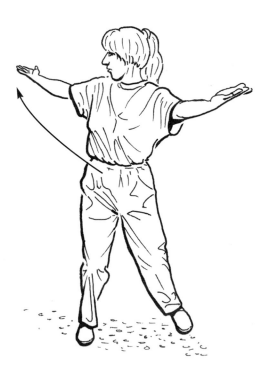

- Your knees bend slightly as the hand drops level with your thigh, then straighten slightly as your hand ascends behind you. Your torso will naturally rotate to the right, but ensure the movement comes from rotating the spine, thus minimizing any turning from the hip.

As you exhale

- Bring your right hand forward in a line so that your thumb passes within 4–6 in. (10–15 cm) of your ear.

- Your right hand continues forward and your right palm comes to face downward towards your left palm, which has turned to face upward.

- The left hand then descends downward on your next inhalation as the cycle repeats itself on the left side.

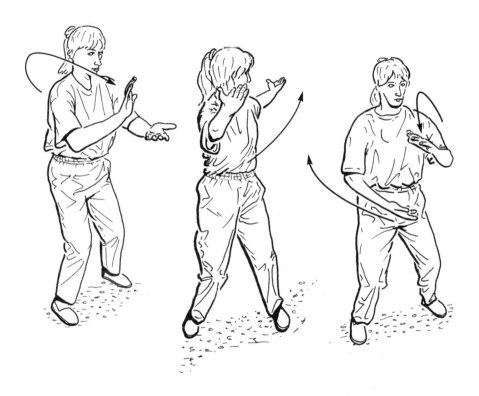

Note

- As in all twisting movements, initiate the movement from your waist. Keep your eyes fixed on the moving hand at all times. Imagine each P-8 point is an eye that wants to keep the other one in sight. Thus the wrists subtly turn throughout the movement to maintain this connection.

■ Mental Focus

Basic Focus

- Focus your attention on Laogong (Pericardium-8), feeling that there is a constant plasma-like connection of Qi between both palms. Use natural breathing (page 58).

Intermediate Focus

- Simply imagine you are extending Qi way beyond your hands as you move them. In other words, the arcs you are making with your hands seem like much bigger arcs, not limited by the length of your arms.

■ Internal Effects

The twisting of your entire body along its vertical axis unblocks and disperses Qi within the Liver and Gall Bladder channels, which are situated mostly on the sides of your body (Figures 12 and 13, page 23). The fact that your hands sweep past your hip on the way back and past the side of your head on the way forward will mildly enhance the dispersing effect upon the Gall Bladder channel in those areas.

■ Benefits

Helps alleviate temporal headaches, migraine and pain in the eyes because ...

- Blockage of Qi in the Gall Bladder channel in the head will lead to temporal headache. Qi in the Liver and Gall Bladder channels tends to rise to the head if it is agitated or not flowing smoothly. This can cause migraine. Both the Liver and Gall Bladder channels have deep connections directly with the eyes, so calming those channels can "calm" pain in the eyes.

6

Rowing a Boat
(...in the Middle of a Lake)

■ Stance and Movements

Simple Version

(The arm movements of this exercise resemble the butterfly swimming stroke).

As you conclude the previous exercise, bring your hands down by your sides and turn your palms outward.

As you inhale

- Circle your arms out to the sides and up above your head.

As you exhale

- Bend your knees, bringing your arms forward and down, inclining your torso slightly forward, keeping your back straight.

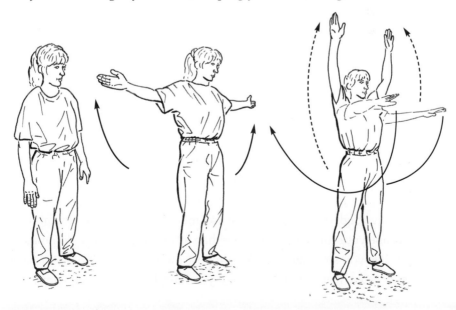

As you inhale

- Straighten your knees and torso while again circling your arms outward and overhead.

More Dynamic Version

(This version is essentially the same as the simple version, except that you exaggerate the bending of your torso and knees, and sort of 'throw your arms away' as if they are loose, lifeless appendages. (A very complicated one to illustrate, so, look at the pictures carefully!)

As you inhale

- Circle your arms out to the sides and up above your head.

As you exhale strongly through your mouth

- Bend your knees and throw your arms forward and down, inclining your torso forward.

- The momentum of your arms will carry them behind you and naturally out to the sides before they end up ahead of you with the backs of your hands facing each other. This will only work if your shoulders and arms are 100% relaxed and limp.

As you slowly inhale

- Unfurl your torso back to the upright position, with your arms hanging down.

- Straighten your knees as you do so.

- Continue the same inhalation and bring your arms again out to the sides and above your head.

Proceed with repetitions without breaking the flow.

Note

- If you have high or low blood pressure, follow the simple version and do not incline your torso forward more than 90 degrees, because you might faint when you straighten up. Also, follow the simple version if you have recently eaten, feel a bit delicate, or if you have lower back problems.

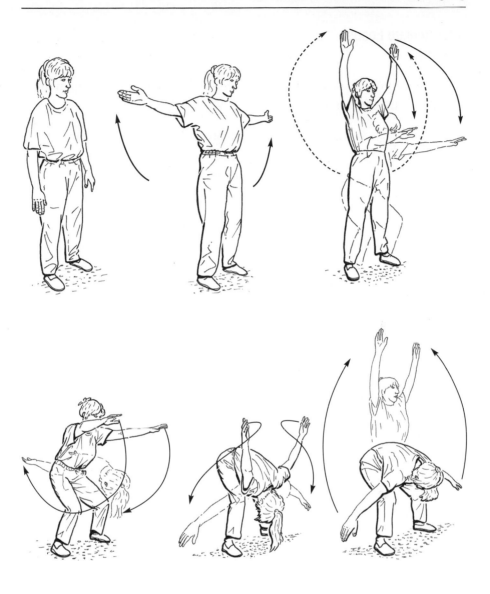

■ Mental Focus

Basic Focus

- Focus your attention on Laogong (Pericardium-8).

- Use natural breathing (page 58).

Intermediate Focus
Option 1

- Imagine you are standing firmly rooted in the sand, ankle deep in the surf on the seashore.

- As you raise your arms, feel that you are pulling in the entire ocean through Yongquan (Kidney-1) in the soles of your feet, sucking it up into your kidneys (but don't lose that feeling of your Qi descending downward through your feet at the same time).

- As you lower your arms, the water drains out through your feet. Meanwhile, feel that you have retained the unlimited power (kinetic energy) of the ocean, which has transformed any fear, apprehension, or timidity.

Option 2

- When your hands are raised, extend Qi through your hands and feel you are connecting with the vastness of space, and become "one" with Heaven Qi.

- When your hands are down, extend Qi through your hands and feet deep into the ground and feel yourself connect and become "one" with Earth Qi.

- After a few repetitions, you will feel that you are drawing Heaven Qi through your body into the earth, and pulling Earth Qi through your body into the sky.

Advanced Focus

- Use the single breath reverse breathing cycle (page 72).

- Sometimes it is good to use the heel raising option to facilitate this focus, i.e., raise your heels as you inhale and gently sink your heels back down as you exhale.

■ Internal Effects

Positive Qi may naturally supplement your Small Circulation. Any emotional and physical tensions will transform into free flowing Qi (*see* A Note About Internal Effects, page 73).

■ Benefits

Excellent for kidney and bladder function because …

- The connotations and imagery of this exercise largely center around water, and water is most closely associated with the kidneys and bladder.

- All exercises where you bend forward then straighten up, such as the more dynamic version of this exercise, stretch and compress the physical kidneys, helping the circulation of blood through them, as well as regulating the kidney's water filtering aspect.

- The forward bending aspect stretches your Bladder channel, much of which runs down the back of your torso (*see* Figure 8, page 22).

Helps balance the peripheral and autonomic nervous systems, leading to a better ability to **combat the effects of stress because …**

- The Bladder channel in your back, because of its proximity to the spine, has an influence on the peripheral nerve roots and the autonomic nerve roots, which themselves are closely connected with the spine.

- The adrenal glands, which are located on top of the kidneys, control adrenalin and other hormones. Like the kidneys, these glands also benefit from the body bending forward and straightening up.

7

Lifting the Ball (sometimes called "Holding a Ball in Front of the Shoulders")

■ Stance and Movements

(This exercise has a rather "statuesque" appearance, rather resembling a thespian proudly presenting a precious jewel (i.e., the ball) in the palm of their hand to an audience).

After straightening up from the previous exercise, inhale and

- Turn 45 degrees to the left and shift your weight to your left foot.

- Lift your right arm diagonally in front of your body until your right palm is slightly higher than your left shoulder. Your palm faces upward. Meanwhile your left hand moves outward. For an added nuance, you could also move that lower hand slightly back so that your left LI-4 (Hegu) point is level with your left GB-30 (Huantiao) point.

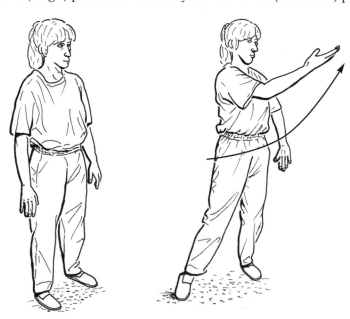

- As you raise your right arm, allow your right heel to lift off the floor. As an optional extra, you can tap the big toe of your right foot against the ground.

As you exhale back to center

- Equalize the weight between both legs and bring the right arm back to your right side. Some practitioners prefer to turn their palms to face down as the arm is lowered, while others prefer to keep the palm facing up. Experiment and feel what gives you the strongest sense of Qi in your hands. It may change from day to day.

- Immediately shift your weight to your right leg and repeat the exercise by raising your left hand.

Note

- Keep your eyes constantly fixed upon the hand that is being raised and lowered. Feeling that you are proudly presenting your 'ball' will encourage a subtle opening of chest and lengthening of spine, which will increase the power of the exercise (*see* Internal Effects, page 73, and Benefits, page 76).

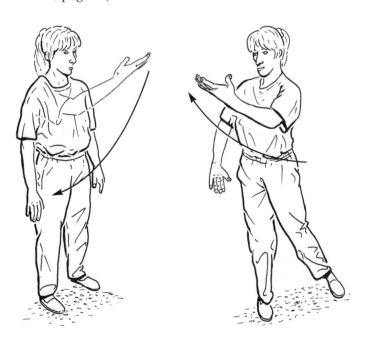

■ Mental Focus

Basic Focus

- Focus your attention on Laogong (Pericardium-8).

- Use natural breathing (page 58).

Intermediate Focus
Option 1

- As you raise your right hand, feel a connection between the Laogong point and your right big toe. Feel the connection as an elastic fiber that stretches as your hand rises, but which must be anchored by rooting the big toe firmly into the ground.

- At the same time, you will feel the weight shift to your left foot, so extend Qi through that foot to deeply connect with Earth Qi.

- Similarly, when you lift your left hand, connect the left Laogong point to your left big toe and extend Qi through your right foot.

Option 2

- Visualize a wave of Qi washing up the right side of your whole body and head as you raise your right hand. As you lower the hand, feel the Qi wash down the right side of your whole body and head.

■ Internal Effects

By pressing the big toe into the floor, the movement of this exercise tonifies the Spleen channel (*see* Figure 5, page 22). It also encourages an awareness of Qi and the free flow of Qi through the Middle Mai.

■ Benefits

This exercise specifically strengthens your body's ability to hold your organs and other soft structures in place, which is a function ascribed to the

Spleen in Chinese medicine. In other words it **helps prevent the prolapse of internal organs and structures and varicose veins, because …**

- There is a strong sense of internal "lift" as you do this exercise, which you can clearly feel, which does not contradict the strong sense of grounding that is felt simultaneously. This feeling is an experiential effect of the Spleen's lifting and holding quality.

Gives you a greater sense of presence because …

- The attitude of the posture is synonymous with boldness and presence.

- The activation of the Spleen's lifting and holding function has a psychological reflection, so that you feel supported and more "uplifted" in spirit.

8

(Turning to...) Gaze at the Moon

■ Stance and Movements

Stand as if you are holding a ball in front of your pelvis.

As you inhale

- Shift your weight into your left leg and swivel your torso to the left. At the same time lift your arms out to the side and up, as if you are looking at the moon and holding your view of the moon between your hands. Lifting your right heel will give you a greater sense of bodily lengthening, especially around your waist and right leg. Keeping your right heel on the ground will increase the rotation of your spinal joints. The choice is yours.

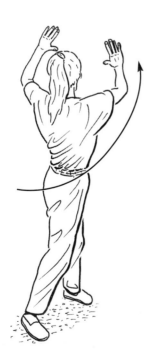
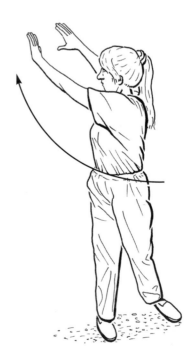

As you exhale

- Bring your hands down in front of your pelvis, equalizing the weight through both legs and bending your knees a little.

- Repeat on the other side by inhaling as you shift your weight into your right leg and lift your arms up to the right.

■ Mental Focus

Basic Focus

- Focus your attention on Laogong (Pericardium-8), trying to keep a strong Qi connection between both palms. When the hands are up, imagine you are looking at the moon as you hold the moon's silhouette between your hands.

- Use natural breathing (page 58).

Intermediate Focus

- Similar to Exercise 7, as you raise hands up and to the left, feel a connection between both palms and your right big toe, and extend Qi into the ground through your left foot. Feel the hand-toe connection as an elastic fiber that stretches as your hands rise, but which must be anchored by rooting the big toe firmly into the ground. Similarly connect your hands to your left big toe when you raise your hands to the right, extending Qi downward through your right foot.

■ Internal Effects

The movement of this exercise tonifies the Spleen channel (*see* Figure 5, page 22). The Liver and Gall Bladder channels are slightly stretched, which moves and smooths their flow of Qi (*see* Figures 12 and 13, page 23). It also supports the upward movement of Qi through the Middle Mai.

■ Benefits

This exercise has similar, but slightly less powerful, "lifting and holding" benefits as Exercise 7.

9

(Turning Waist and...) Pushing Palm

■ Stance and Movements

Adopt a well-rooted basic stance and hold loose upturned fists next to your waist.

As you inhale

- Turn your torso diagonally to the left as you extend your right hand in front of you and your left hand backward and downward. During this phase, your palms open out as your wrists rotate inward: the right wrist rotates so that the palm ends up facing forward with the fingertips pointing up. The left wrist rotates so that the palm faces downward with fingertips pointing forward.

As you exhale

- Rotate the wrists outward as you close the palms, so they arrive face up next to your waist as your torso faces forward.

As you inhale

- Turn to the right and perform a mirror image of the movement on that side.

Variation

Instead of bringing your fists back to your sides each time you exhale, cross your hands, palms up in front of Dantian. Whichever hand is about to stretch forward should be the one on top.

Note

- Keep both feet flat on the ground throughout, even though you may be tempted to raise your heels. Also, ensure the knees do not drift toward each other.

- Inhale when you extend your arm forward, even though it may initially feel more natural to exhale (which will be the case if you do a martial art where exhaling as you punch is the norm).

- When your hand extends forward and opens, lead with the thumb and index finger side of your hand. This will activate LI-4 (Hegu) and animate the Large Intestine channel. Do the same with the hand that is pressing backward and downward.

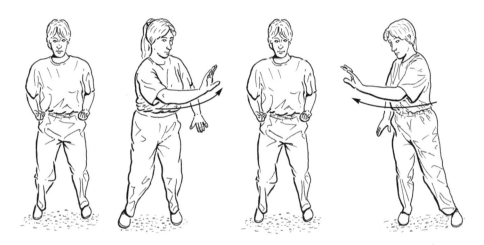

■ Mental Focus

Basic Focus

- Focus on Laogong of the palm that is pressed forward.

- Use natural breathing (page 58).

Intermediate Focus

- As you inhale and extend one arm forward, imagine a beam of Qi (perhaps visualized as a beam of light or an elastic cord) connecting LI-4 (Hegu) with your Lower Dantian or if preferred, your Middle Dantian.

- As you exhale and retract your arms, focus your mind on Laogong.

- It may also be helpful to feel that Laogong on the hand—which is going backward and downward during inhalation—is compressing a springy ball of Qi, which fills the space between your palm and the floor.

■ Internal Effects

Inhaling with reverse abdominal breathing as your arms move forward causes Qi to move from the surface of the limbs directly inward toward the bones. Then, during the exhalation phase, Qi moves from the interior of the limbs to the surface, thus strengthening the Qi that protects you from pathogenic factors entering via the surface of your body. This Qi is known as Defensive Qi (Wei Qi). The Source of Defensive Qi is further strengthened as a result of the strong stimulation of Qi in the Lower and Middle Dantian (see Original Qi, page 17).

■ Benefits

Aids digestion and regulates bowel movement because ...

- This exercise very effectively moves Qi in your Lower Dantian (affecting the bowels, and to some extent the bladder) or Middle Dantian (affecting the stomach and digestive process), depending on your focus.

- The position of the hands strongly opens and tonifies the Large Intestine channel which runs from your index finger, up the back of your arm, over the top of your shoulder and into your face, at the base of your nostril.

Helps build resistance to cold or hot weather, wind, and other external influences because ...

- The Defensive Qi is strengthened.

10

Hands in Cloud (...in Horse Stance)

■ Stance and Movements

As you perform the final repetition of Exercise 9, your left hand will be outstretched in front of you and your right hand pressed down behind you. From there, turn your left palm to face you and raise it to eye level. Bring your right hand forward in front of your waist with the palm facing toward your left.

As you inhale

- Turn your head and torso to the left, keeping your eyes fixed on your raised hand. Your lower hand remains held a few inches from Dantian as you turn. In other words, you move your torso, arms, and head as a single unit.

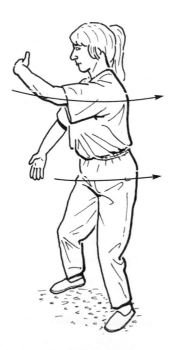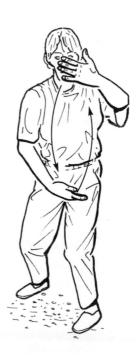

- Having turned about 45 degrees to your left, raise your right palm to eye level. Simultaneously lower the left hand to waist level, with the palm facing your left.

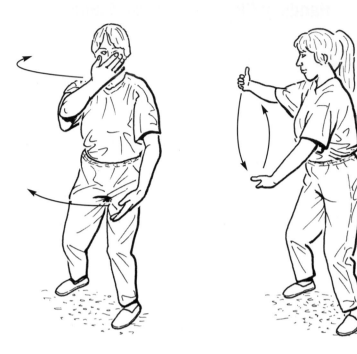

As you exhale

- Turn your head, torso, and arms to the right as you exhale. When you reach 45 degrees right, switch the hands again and inhale back to the left.

Variations

Although the position of the lower hand is traditionally described as facing to the left or right, some practitioners find that turning the palm down works well. Others find that turning the lower palm up is effective. Once you have some experience, play around with your hand position to see what gives you the clearest experience of Qi in your hands.

A less common—but equally valid variation—is to have the palm of the upper hand turned away from your face, so that you are looking at the back of your hand. Having the upper palm turned away can have a slightly cooling and "clearing out" effect, whereas palm turned toward you has a more warming and "containing" nuance.

Note

- Breathe in as you turn to the left and exhale as you turn to the right. Make all aspects of the movement and the connection between repetitions of the exercise a seamless continuum. The movement should be led by the turning movement of the waist, and therefore not led by the arms. When looking at your raised palm, gently relax your gaze on the spaces between your fingers. There are two distinct methods of weight shifting the legs, (1) keep equal weight through both legs when turning, (2) weight shift into the left leg when turning to the left and into the right leg when turning to the right.

■ Mental Focus

Basic Focus

- Be aware of Laogong in each palm. Imagine there is a vertical column of Qi connecting your hands, which moves around a vertical axis, i.e., your spine.

Intermediate Focus

- While gently resting your gaze on the spaces between your fingers, see if you can let go of your eye's tendency to focus. Eventually you should see a narrow shadowy outline around the silhouette of your fingers.

■ Internal Effects

During this exercise, the spine is rotating perfectly through its neutral and vertically aligned position. This helps "open" the Back Mai.

■ Benefits

Cleanses the eyes. Calms the mind by relaxing the eyes because ...

- Consciousness is influenced by stimuli received through the eyes. (Try relaxing while watching some frenetic or violent activity!)

11

Scooping the Sea (...and Viewing the Sky)

■ Stance and Movements

Bring your left foot forward to adopt a bow stance, i.e., your back foot turns out to 45 degrees and your front foot faces forward, or if preferred, angled very slightly inward. The forward leg is bent at the knee while the back leg is straight. This is the traditional posture for shooting arrows from a bow. Cross your hands in front of your left knee with your right hand in front.

As you inhale

- Shift your weight into your back foot, so that the back knee bends a little and the front knee straightens. At the same time, bring your arms overhead and separate them, looking slightly upward at the sky (or ceiling) as you do so.

As you exhale

- Tilt your body forward by shifting your weight from back foot to front foot, naturally lowering both arms by your sides to again cross at your knee. Look at your hands when in this position.

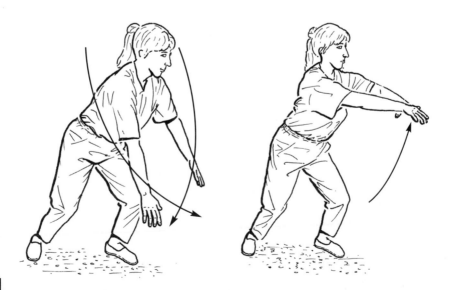

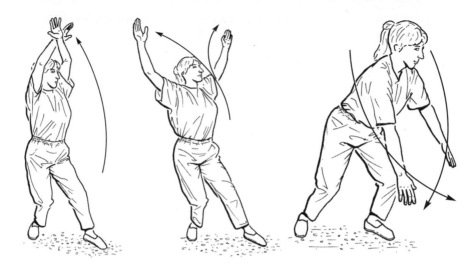

Note

* Keep both feet flat on the ground throughout. When looking at the sky, don't overdo it by craning back your neck. Instead, try to keep a sense of lengthening and "opening" at the back of your neck and of your spine as a whole.

■ Mental Focus

Basic Focus

* Focus your attention on Laogong (Pericardium-8).

* Use natural breathing (page 58).

Intermediate Focus
Option 1
If you are feeling "full" and "blocked" and want to dissolve or transform this fullness or blockage of Qi:

* As you raise your arms and inhale, imagine clear water (if you feel hot) or warm fine sand (if you feel cold) is being sucked up through Yongquan (Kidney-1) into your legs and filling your entire body, absorbing and transforming the tensions, stress, pain, anger, etc.

* As you lower your arms and exhale, feel the water or sand flood out through the soles of your feet and deep into the earth, to be replaced with fresh water or sand during your next inhalation.

- Use natural or normal breathing. You can also use reverse breathing if proficient.

Option 2
If you are feeling "empty" and listless and want to absorb fresh Qi:

- Imagine you are enveloped within a ball of pure white light or fluid-like nectar which you absorb as you do the movements.

Option 3
If you are feeling isolated or "disconnected":

- Extend Qi as far as possible from your hands so that when they go up, your Qi connects with Heaven Qi. Meanwhile, extend Qi downward through your back foot, feeling a connection with Earth Qi.

- When your hands come down, your Qi connects deeply with Earth Qi by extending Qi out from your hands and downward through your front foot. This will produce a strong sensation of "connection" between yourself and all the elements around you.

Advanced Focus

- Use the single breath reverse breathing cycle (page 72).

■ Internal Effects

Heaven Qi and Earth Qi may naturally supplement your Small Circulation. Any emotional and physical tensions will transform into free flowing Qi (*see* A Note About Internal Effects, page 73).

■ Benefits

Opens and expands Qi in the chest, thereby strengthening the heart and lungs which **helps reduce depression, because ...**

- The heart affects, and is most affected by, joy/excitement.

- The lung affects, and is most affected by, grief/depression.

12

Pushing Waves (sometimes called "Playing With Waves" or "Reinforcing Waves")

■ Stance and Movements

The bow stance and leg movements are the same as Exercise 11 except you raise your

- Back heel when you lean forward;

- Front toes by pivoting on the heel when you lean back.

Take your weight on your back foot and inhale as you

- Raise your arms to shoulder height, palms down.

- Bring your hands back to within about 4 in. (10 cm) of your chest, turning your palms slightly forward as you do so.

As you exhale

- Shift your weight to your front foot, straightening your back leg and bending your front leg, as you;

- Extend your arms forward, palms facing the front; as if you're pushing the waves away.

Inhale again as you

- Lean into your back foot and bring your hands back toward your chest again.

Hence the cycle repeats itself as you again exhale and extend your arms.

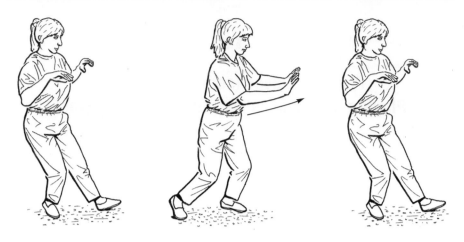

Variation

Rather than bend your front leg when shifting weight into it, keep it straight instead. This will result in a slight lift up the front of your body when moving forward, which will slightly "open" your Stomach and Spleen channels.

Note

• Keep your spine, head, and neck in vertical alignment throughout.

■ Mental Focus

Basic Focus

• Focus your attention on Laogong (Pericardium-8). Use natural breathing (page 58).

• Imagine you are pulling the sea toward you when you inhale and pull back. Imagine you are pushing the sea away from you as you exhale and extend forward.

Intermediate Focus

• As you pull the sea toward you, feel yourself firmly standing your ground as the wave washes through you, loosening, cooling, and transforming your tensions and anxieties; or if you prefer, dragging tensions and anxieties out through the back of your body.

• Then as you push your arms forward, imagine the wave that passed through you return through your back and complete the cooling and transforming process; or if you prefer, wash out more tension through the front of your body.

- After a few repetitions, you could switch your intention to absorbing the power of the sea as you draw it in and push it out. You could imagine that wave power is charging up your kidneys rather like a wave-powered hydroelectricity generator.

- If you also extend Qi through your feet as each one in turn takes the weight, this exercise becomes even more effective, because it adds to the sense of "standing your ground."

Advanced Focus

- Use the single breath reverse breathing cycle (page 72).

■ Internal Effects

Heaven Qi and Earth Qi may naturally supplement your Small Circulation. Any emotional and physical tensions will transform into free flowing Qi (*see* A Note About Internal Effects, page 73).

■ Benefits

Excellent for kidney and bladder function because …

- The connotations and imagery of this exercise largely center around water, and water is most closely associated with the kidneys and bladder.

Efficiently transforms or expels tensions and anxieties because …

- The imagery of cleansing with water is extremely powerful within this exercise.

Gives you the ability to "stand your ground" or manifest your will because …

- The imagery of absorbing the latent power of the ocean is very strong. The power of the ocean represents the most powerful energy on the planet; able even to erode continents. Once it is on the move (tidal movement) nothing can stop it.

13

Flying Dove (...Spreads its Wings)

■ Stance and Movements

This exercise has exactly the same stance and leg movements as Exercise 12.

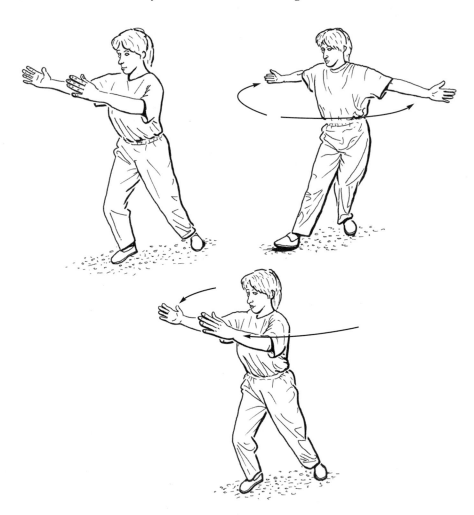

As you inhale

- Adopt a bow stance with the weight on your back foot, opening your arms out to the sides with your palms facing forward.

As you exhale

- Move forward, bringing your weight onto your front foot as you close your arms ahead of you, so that P-8 (Laogong) in both palms come within a few centimeters of each other.

- Again, lean weight into your back foot as you open your arms on an inhalation.

Note

- Keep your spine, head, and neck in vertical alignment throughout.

■ Mental Focus

Basic Focus

- Focus your attention on Laogong (Pericardium-8).

- Use natural breathing (page 58).

Intermediate Focus

- As you open your arms, hold the image and feeling of pulling Qi out of the Middle Dantian with your palms via Shanzhong (Ren-17) to spiral open into a large bubble of Qi in front of your chest.

- At the same time, you will feel the weight shift to your back foot, so extend Qi through that foot to deeply connect with Earth Qi.

- If you feel like distributing some positive Qi in the form of compassion or goodwill toward others, let the Qi bubble disperse and radiate to all beings. If you have some anger, grief, or other such emotions, you can hold the idea that those emotions are within your Qi bubble, to be transformed by the neutrality of a surrounding Universal Qi.

- Gather in your Qi bubble (imbued with fresh Qi) when closing your arms.

- After a few repetitions, you might be able to imagine a sky-blue light ascend from the Lower Dantian to the Middle Dantian as you begin to step back and open your arms.

Advanced Focus

- Use the single breath reverse breathing cycle (page 72).

■ Internal Effects

Heaven Qi and Earth Qi may naturally supplement your Small Circulation. Any emotional and physical tensions will transform into free flowing Qi (*see* A Note About Internal Effects, page 73).

■ Benefits

Opens and expands Qi in the chest, thereby strengthening the heart and lungs which **helps reduce depression, because the ...**

- Heart affects, and is most affected by, joy/excitement.

- Lung affects, and is most affected by, grief/depression.

14

Charging Fists (...With Outstretched Arms)

■ Stance and Movements

Stand with your feet hip-width apart and parallel, clench fists and place them beside your waist, palm side up.

As you inhale

- Slowly punch your right fist forward, rotating it on the way so that the closed palm faces down. The arm and hand should be relaxed throughout and the elbow should just fall short of locking out straight.

As you exhale

- Withdraw your fist, rotating it on the way so that the palm side faces up.

- Repeat with the left fist. Thereafter alternating fists with each inhalation.

Variation

As your fist reaches its most forward position after fully inhaling, retain the breath and tense the arm muscles without tensing the fist or shoulders. If you get this right, it will feel like the muscles of your arm and forearm "grip" around the bones. Fully relax the arm as you retract it on an exhalation.

Note

- Try not to let your elbow bow out to the side when punching forward or retracting the fist. Punching forward can also be done during an exhalation rather than an inhalation. The exhalation option opens the joints in the arm and shoulder more. The inhalation option builds Qi more effectively.

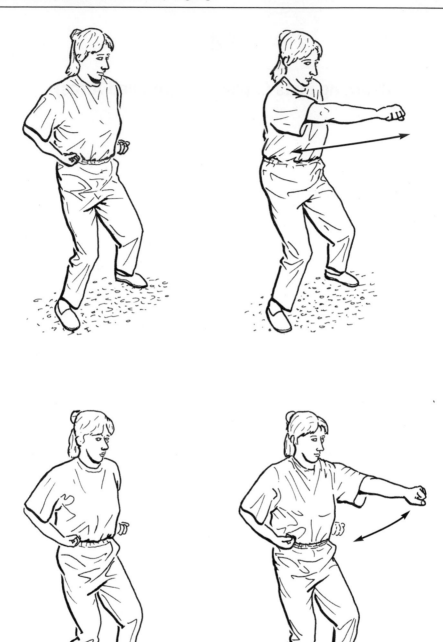

■ Mental Focus

Basic Focus

- Focus your attention on Laogong (Pericardium-8). Use natural breathing (page 58).

Intermediate Focus

- Imagine an elastic plasma like Qi connection between your fists and your Lower Dantian, that is stretched as your fist moves forward.

- Experiment with normal (page 63) and reverse abdominal breathing (page 62) and notice the different sensations this gives within your belly.

■ Internal Effects

Inhaling with reverse abdominal breathing as your arms move forward causes Qi to move from the surface of the limbs directly inward toward the bones. During the exhalation phase, Qi moves from the interior of the limbs to the surface, thus strengthening the Defensive Qi that protects you from pathogenic factors entering via the surface of your body. The source of Defensive Qi is further strengthened as a result of the strong stimulation of Qi in the Lower and Middle Dantians (*see* Original Qi, page 17).

■ Benefits

Aids digestion and regulates bowel movement because ...

- This exercise very effectively moves Qi in your Lower Dantian (affecting the bowels, and to some extent the bladder) or Middle Dantian (affecting the stomach and digestive process), depending on your focus.

Helps build resistance to cold or hot weather, wind, and other external influences because ...

- The Defensive Qi is strengthened.

15

Flying Wild Goose

■ Stance and Movements

Stand in the basic stance with your arms out to the side parallel to the ground, at shoulder height, palms down. Inhale.

As you exhale

- Bend your knees and sink deeper into your stance as you lower your arms like graceful wings. Some people cross their forearms when the arms are down, which feels good.

As you inhale

- Raise your stance a little and unfurl your arms out to the sides, in a graceful "spreading of wings" manner.

Note

- The wrists should feel very pliable as your arms move. Your arms should have a very relaxed and malleable wave-like quality throughout.

■ Mental Focus

Basic Focus

- Focus your attention on Laogong (Pericardium-8).

- Use natural breathing (page 58).

Intermediate Focus
Option 1

- As you raise your arms up like spreading wings, feel that you are unfurling much larger wings of Qi which stretch for great distances either side of you. As they do so, they absorb Heaven Qi in the form of light and air.

- As you lower your "wings of Qi," they sweep into the ground to absorb Earth Qi.

Option 2
If you are feeling "full" or "blocked," and want to eliminate "negative" Qi:

- As you raise your arms and inhale, imagine clear water (if you feel hot) or warm fine sand (if you feel cold) is being sucked up through Yongquan (Kidney-1) into your legs and filling your entire body, absorbing and transforming the tensions, stress, pain, anger, etc.

- As you lower your arms and exhale, feel the water or sand flood out through the soles of your feet and deep into the earth, to be replaced with fresh water or sand during your next inhalation.

- Throughout this exercise, remember that when you raise your arms, feel your Qi descend from your Lower Dantian into the ground to meet with and absorb Earth Qi. As such, you should adopt natural or normal breathing so that Ren-1 (Huiyin) opens as your arms are raised during inhalation.

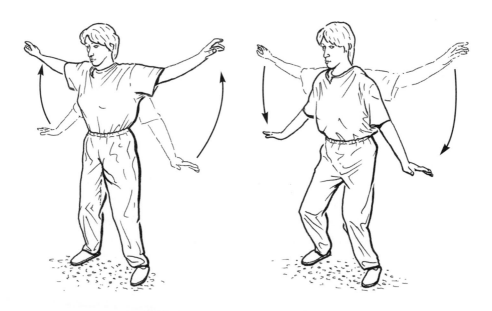

Option 3

If you are feeling "empty" and listless and want to absorb fresh Qi:

- Imagine you are enveloped within a ball of pure white light or fluid-like nectar which you absorb as you do the movements.

Advanced Focus
Option 1

- Use the single breath reverse breathing cycle (page 72).

- Sometimes it is good to use the heel raising option to facilitate this focus, i.e., raise your heels as you inhale and gently sink your heels back down as you exhale.

Option 2

- Using normal or reverse abdominal breathing, as you raise your arms to the side, visualize a sky-blue light traveling from your Lower Dantian up the Middle Mai to your Middle Dantian.

- When your palms reach shoulder height, feel Qi spiraling out of Laogong to open into two large bubbles of Qi, i.e., one beyond each set of fingertips. If you feel like distributing some positive Qi in the form of compassion or goodwill toward others, let the Qi bubbles disperse and radiate to all beings. If you have some anger, grief, or other such emotions, you can hold the idea that those emotions are within your Qi bubble, to be transformed by the neutrality of a surrounding Universal Qi.

- After two or three repetitions, gather in fresh Heaven Qi when your arms are up, and Earth Qi when your arms are down.

- As you inhale and raise your arms again, feel that the Qi is pulled into the Middle Mai via the Lower Dantian and raised up as before. In addition, you may like to add to that Qi by drawing in fresh Earth Qi through the soles of your feet.

■ Internal Effects

Heaven Qi and Earth Qi may naturally supplement your Small Circulation. Any emotional and physical tensions will transform into free flowing Qi (*see* A Note About Internal Effects, page 73).

■ Benefits

Opens and expands Qi in the chest, particularly strengthening the lungs which **helps reduce depression and feelings of isolation, because ...**

- The lungs affect, and are most affected by, grief/depression.

- The lungs relate to your sense of boundary. If your Lung Qi is weak, you may find it difficult to allow people into your "space." You may also have difficulty moving out of your space or crossing boundaries into other spaces. Thus, you may become depressed through isolation. This is actually a great exercise to do if a feeling of loneliness is sapping your will to practice the other exercises.

16

Spinning Wheel

■ Stance and Movements

Stand with knees slightly bent in the basic stance. Bend forward with palms facing the ground, head, and neck relaxed.

As you inhale

- Straighten your arms and from your waist, circle your torso and arms to the left and up, straightening your legs a little as you do so.

- Keep your palms turned out, as if you are using them to wipe the inside of a huge wheel.

As you exhale

- Continue circling to the right and down, bending your knees as your arms drop.

- At the bottom of the circle, swing slightly beyond the centerline to the left.

As you inhale

- Swing back to the right and up.

Note

- Look at your hands throughout the movement. Some practitioners keep their legs straight while circling, but to do so risks injuring the lumbar vertebral discs, so it is not recommended. Lead the movement from the Lower Dantian, i.e., initiate it from the waist, so that the arms follow rather than lead the movement.

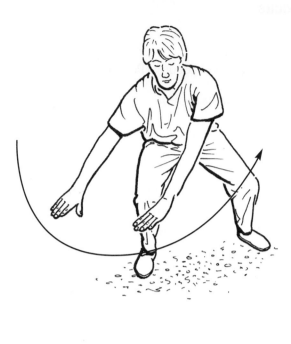

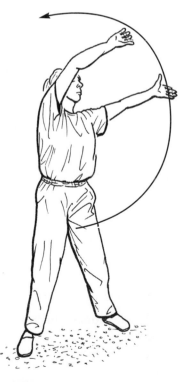

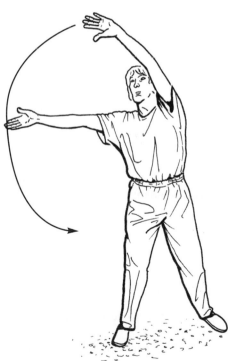

■ Mental Focus

Basic Focus

- Focus your attention on Laogong (Pericardium-8).

- Use natural breathing (page 58).

Intermediate Focus
Option 1

- If you need to really move yourself because you feel "bottled up," you can do this exercise with some speed, so that centrifugal force moves your Qi and blood; transforming it from stagnation to a free flowing state. If you like the concept of expelling rather than transforming, hold the image of tension and anxieties being flung out through your palms and fingertips.

Option 2

- Extend Qi as far as you can through your hands as you move them, feeling that as they go up they connect with Heaven Qi, and as they go down they connect through the ground with Earth Qi. Hence, the exercise gives a strong sense of you melding with and integrating all the positive energies around you.

■ Internal Effects

Strongly moves Qi and blood to your hands. Also, the circular movement smoothes the Qi in all the channels by dispersing any stagnation of Qi in the Liver and Gall Bladder channels (*see* Figures 12 and 13, page 23). A function of the Liver in Chinese medicine is the "smoothing" of Qi flow in general.

■ Benefits

Improves vitality by stimulating the elimination of waste products because ...

- Circling from the waist facilitates bowel and liver function.

- Circling downward and back up flushes the kidneys.

17

Bouncing a Ball (...While Stepping)

■ Stance and Movements

Stand relaxed and upright, with arms hanging loosely by your sides.

As you inhale

- Shift your weight into your right foot and slowly lift your left leg, allowing it to bend at the knee (keeping foot and ankle relaxed).

- Simultaneously raise your right hand so that it reaches just above shoulder height at the same time as the left knee reaches hip height.

- The wrist is totally relaxed so that the fingertips point toward the ground.

As you exhale

- Slowly and simultaneously lower your hand and leg. The foot should touch the ground at the same time as the hand reaches its lowest position.

- As the arm descends, the palm should angle forward, as if you are gently stroking something.

Repeat on the other side, alternating sides with each inhalation (a bit like marching through treacle)!

Variation

When your hand is fully raised, you could give it a little flick, as if bouncing a ball; either as you retain the breath between inhaling and exhaling, or at the beginning of your exhalation. This is a good option if your wrists are stiff (because Qi has stagnated in your wrists).

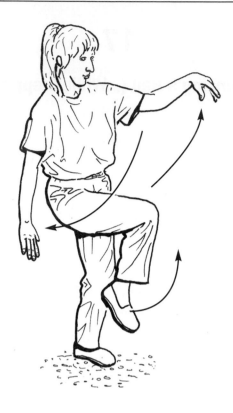

Note

- Look straight ahead throughout.

■ Mental Focus

Basic Focus

- Focus your attention on Laogong (Pericardium-8).

- Use natural breathing (page 58).

Intermediate Focus

- As you raise your hand, feel a "chord-like" connection of Qi between Laogong in your palm and Yongquan (Kidney-1) on the sole of your rising foot. (Hence the hand and foot become one in movement.)

- At the same time, you will feel the weight shift to your other foot, so extend Qi through that foot to deeply connect with Earth Qi.

Advanced Focus

* Use the single breath reverse breathing cycle (page 72).

■ Internal Effects

Heaven Qi and Earth Qi may naturally supplement your Small Circulation. Any emotional and physical tensions will transform into free flowing Qi (*see* A Note About Internal Effects, page 73).

■ Benefits

The unification of movement between your arm and opposite leg increases mental and physical coordination by helping to harmonize the right and left hemispheres of your brain.

18

Calming Qi (sometimes called "Balancing Qi" or "Pressing the Palms for Calming")

■ Stance and Movements

Stand in the basic stance with your palms in front of Dantian, fingers pointing at each other.

As you inhale

- Lift your hands to eye level, allowing the palms to turn toward you slightly.

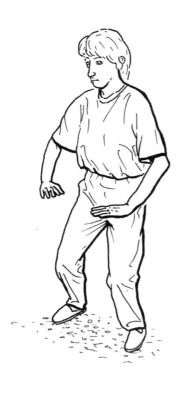 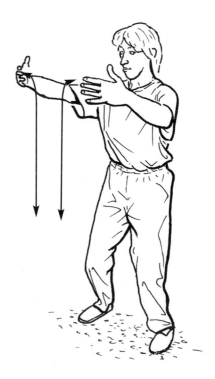

As you exhale

- Turn your palms downward and allow your hands to sink down to Dantian.

- Allow your knees to bend a little as you do so.

Variations

When you inhale and raise your hands, some practitioners like to raise their heels, placing them down again as the hands come down.

Another slight adaptation is to extend your hands forward and up, then backward and down in a circle; rather like using the edge of your little fingers to trace the front and back of a large ball situated in front of your torso.

Note

- It is nice to end this exercise, and therefore the whole set of exercises, by just resting your palms on your lower belly for a few moments; either in standing or sitting. This acts to "close you down" a little, because while performing the exercises, your energy will have opened up to the subtleties of surrounding Qi.

- If you are menstruating, place your hands on your upper belly rather than your lower belly.

■ Mental Focus

Basic Focus

- Focus your attention on Laogong (Pericardium-8). Use natural breathing (page 58).

Intermediate Focus

- As you lower your arms, extend Qi deeply into the ground through Yongquan (Kidney-1) to connect with Earth Qi. At the same time, imagine Heaven Qi is being pulled in through the top of your head and descends through your body into your Lower Dantian.

- Then, as you raise your arms, feel that more Qi descends from your Lower Dantian into the ground to meet with and absorb Earth Qi (which ultimately migrates up into your Lower Dantian).

- After a few repetitions, you should find it natural to experience the melding of Heaven Qi and Earth Qi within your body.

Advanced Focus

- Use the single breath reverse breathing cycle (page 72).

■ Internal Effects

Heaven Qi and Earth Qi may naturally supplement your Small Circulation. Any emotional and physical tensions will transform into free flowing Qi (*see* A Note About Internal Effects, page 73).

■ Benefits

Calms the mind and integrates all the benefits of the previous exercises, because...

- Absorbing the Yin quality of Earth Qi during the rising movement and attracting the Yang quality of Heaven Qi during the descending movement will "negative" you with the Heaven Qi and Earth Qi. This will give you a sense of integration with all things.

Summary of Exercises

All exercises can be performed using the basic focus of holding your attention on Laogong (Pericardium-8) and breathing naturally. Minor additions to this basic focus are given where relevant. One example of an intermediate level of mental focus is given under each exercise described in this section. The advanced focus for most exercises is to use the single breath reverse breathing cycle (page 72).

■ 1. Beginning Movement

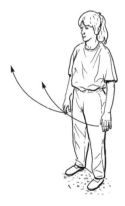 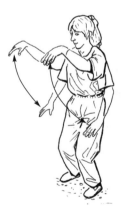

Intermediate Focus

As you lower your arms, connect with Earth Qi by extending Qi through Yongquan (Kidney-1). Then, when you raise your arms, feel that your Qi descends from your Lower Dantian into the ground to meet with and absorb Earth Qi. As such, you should adopt natural breathing, or use normal breathing so that Ren-1 (Huiyin) opens as your arms are raised during inhalation.

■ 2. Opening the Chest

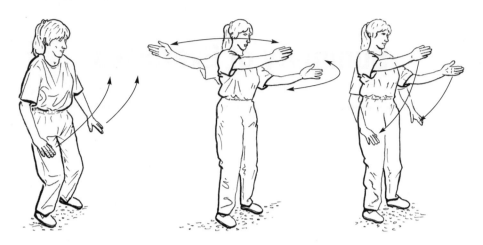

Intermediate Focus

Focus is the same as for Exercise 1.

■ 3. Painting a Rainbow

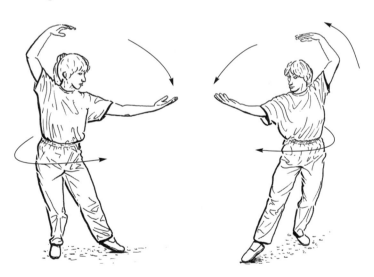

Intermediate Focus

As your hands move from one side to the other, extend Qi through your fingertips, as if you are painting a rainbow with your Qi high in the sky. Simultaneously, extend Qi into the ground through the foot which is taking most weight, and connect your Qi with Earth Qi.

■ 4. Separating the Clouds

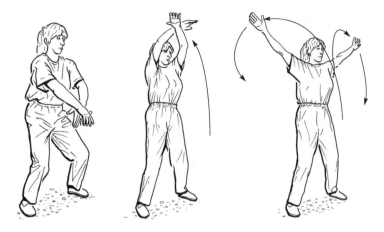

Intermediate Focus

Feel that you are gathering fresh Earth Qi through your feet as you sink your feet into the ground during inhalation. This supportive Earth Qi fills your body, absorbing or transforming any feelings of depression or of being unsupported. As you exhale, Heaven Qi is attracted into your body through the top of your head.

■ 5. Arm Rolling (...in Fixed Stance)

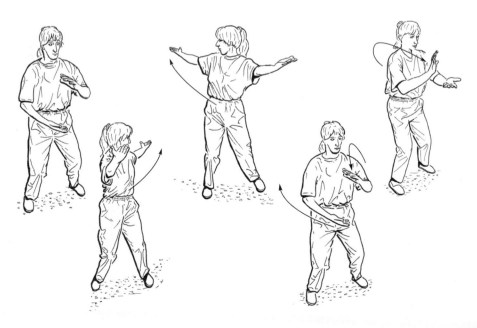

Basic Focus

As you focus your attention on Laogong (Pericardium-8), feel that there is a constant plasma-like connection of Qi between both palms.

Intermediate Focus

Simply imagine you are extending Qi way beyond your hands as you move them. In other words, the arcs you are making with your hands seem like much bigger arcs, not limited by the length of your arms.

■ 6A. Rowing a Boat (...in the Middle of a Lake)

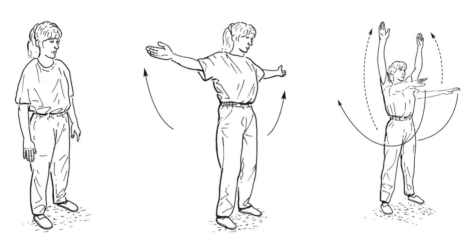

■ 6B. Rowing a Boat (...in the Middle of a Lake)

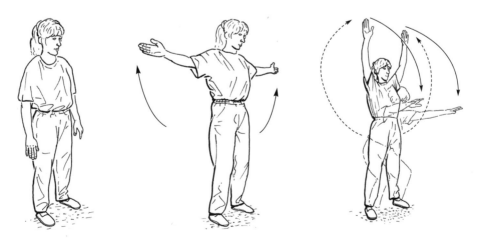

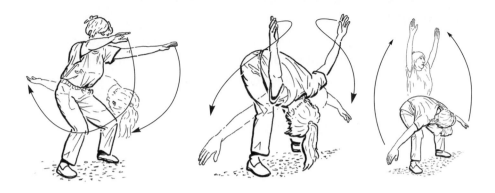

Basic Focus

Focus your attention on Laogong (Pericardium-8) and breathe naturally.

Intermediate Focus

As you raise your arms, feel that you are pulling in the entire ocean through Yongquan (Kidney-1) in the soles of your feet, sucking it up into your kidneys (but don't lose that feeling of your Qi descending downward through your feet at the same time).

As you lower your arms, the water drains out through your feet. Meanwhile, feel that you have retained the unlimited power (kinetic energy) of the ocean, which has transformed any fear, apprehension, or timidity.

■ 7. Lifting the Ball

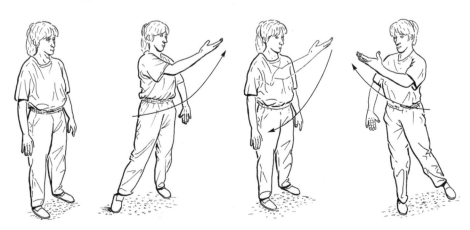

Intermediate Focus

Visualize a wave of Qi washing up the right side of your whole body and head as you raise your right hand. As you lower the hand, feel the Qi wash down the right side of your whole body and head.

■ 8. (Turning to...) Gaze at the Moon

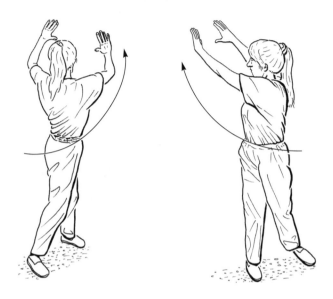

Basic Focus

When your hands are up, imagine you are looking at the moon as you hold the moon's silhouette between your hands.

Intermediate Focus

As you raise hands up and to the left, feel a connection between both palms and your right big toe, and extend Qi into the ground through your left foot. Feel the hand-toe connection as an elastic fiber that stretches as your hands rise, but which must be anchored by rooting the big toe firmly into the ground. Similarly connect your hands to your left big toe when you raise your hands to the right, extending Qi downward through your right foot.

■ 9. (Turning Waist and...) Pushing Palm

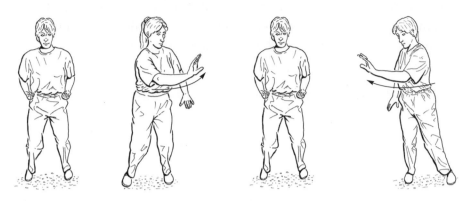

Intermediate Focus

As you inhale and extend one arm forward, imagine a beam of Qi connecting LI-4 (Hegu) with your Lower Dantian or Middle Dantian. As you exhale and retract your arms, focus your mind on Laogong. It may also be helpful to feel that Laogong on the hand which is going backward and downward during inhalation is compressing a springy ball of Qi that fills the space between your palm and the floor.

■ 10. Hands in Cloud (...in Horse Stance)

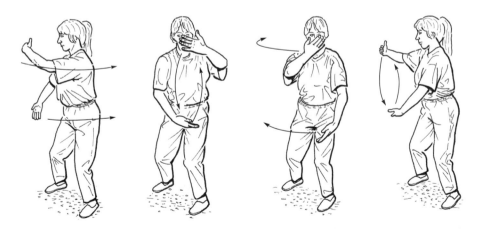

Basic Focus

Be aware of Laogong in each palm. Then imagine there is a vertical column of Qi connecting your hands, which moves around a vertical axis, i.e., your spine.

Intermediate Focus

While gently resting your gaze on the spaces between your fingers, see if you can let go of your eye's tendency to focus. Eventually you should see a narrow shadowy outline around the silhouette of your fingers.

■ 11. Scooping the Sea (...and Viewing the Sky)

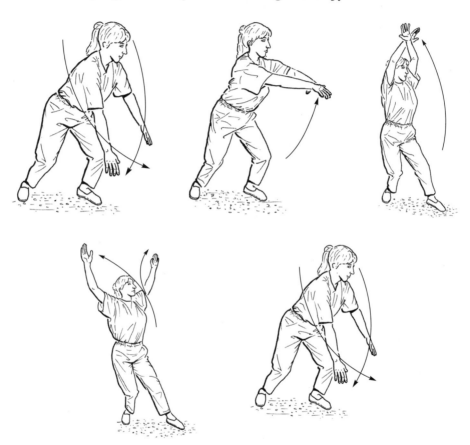

Intermediate Focus

As you raise your arms and inhale, imagine clear water (if you feel hot) or warm fine sand (if you feel cold) is being sucked up through Yongquan (Kidney-1) into your legs and filling your entire body, absorbing and transforming the tensions, stress, pain, anger, etc. As you lower your arms and exhale, feel the water or sand flood out through the soles of your feet and deep into the earth, to be replaced with fresh water or sand during your next inhalation.

■ 12. Pushing Waves

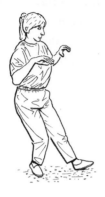 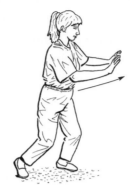 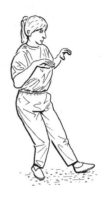

Basic Focus

Imagine you are pulling the sea toward you when you inhale and pull back. Imagine you are pushing the sea away from you as you exhale and extend forward.

Intermediate Focus

As you pull the sea towards you, feel yourself firmly standing your ground as the wave washes through you, loosening, cooling, and transforming your tensions and anxieties. As you push your arms forward, imagine the wave that passed through you returns through your back and completes the cooling and transforming process. After a few repetitions you could switch your intention to absorbing the power of the sea as you draw it in and push it out.

■ 13. Flying Dove (...Spreads its Wings)

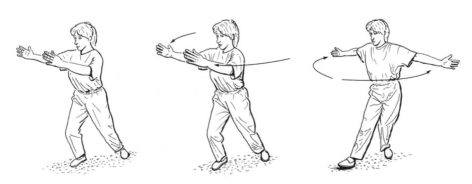

Intermediate Focus

As you open your arms, feel that you are pulling Qi out of Shanzhong (Ren-17) with your palms, to spiral open into a large bubble of Qi in front of your chest. Simultaneously extend Qi through your back foot to deeply connect with Earth Qi. Let the Qi bubble disperse and radiate to all beings. Gather in your Qi bubble (imbued with fresh Qi) when closing your arms.

■ 14. Charging Fists (...With Outstretched Arms)

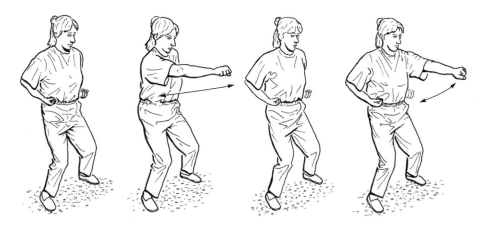

Intermediate Focus

Imagine an elastic plasma-like Qi connection between your fists and your Lower Dantian that is stretched as your fist moves forward.

■ 15. Flying Wild Goose

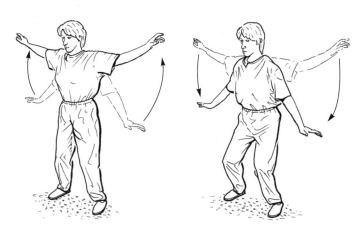

Intermediate Focus

As you raise your arms up like spreading wings, feel that you are unfurling much larger wings of Qi which stretch for great distances either side of you. As they do so, they absorb Heaven Qi in the form of light and air. As you lower your "wings of Qi," they sweep into the ground to absorb Earth Qi.

■ 16. Spinning Wheel

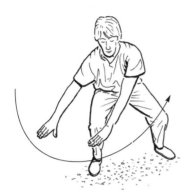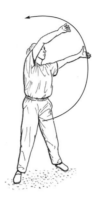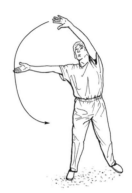

Intermediate Focus

Extend Qi as far as you can through your hands as you move them, feeling that as they go up they connect with Heaven Qi, and as they go down they connect through the ground with Earth Qi. Hence, the exercise gives a strong sense of you melding with and integrating all the positive energies around you.

■ 17. Bouncing a Ball (...While Stepping)

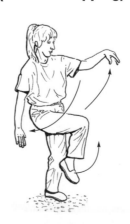

Intermediate Focus

As you raise your hand, feel a "chord-like" connection of Qi between Laogong in your palm and Yongquan (Kidney-1) on the sole of your rising foot. Hence the hand and foot become one in movement. At the same time, you will feel the weight shift to your other foot, so extend Qi through that foot to deeply connect with Earth Qi.

■ 18. Calming Qi

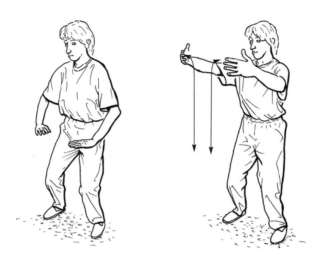

Intermediate Focus

As you lower your arms, extend Qi deeply into the ground through Yongquan (Kidney-1) to connect with Earth Qi. At the same time, imagine Heaven Qi is being pulled in through the top of your head and descends through your body into your Lower Dantian. Then, as you raise your arms, feel that more Qi descends from your Lower Dantian into the ground to meet with and absorb Earth Qi (which ultimately migrates up into your Lower Dantian).

Quick Reference Chart

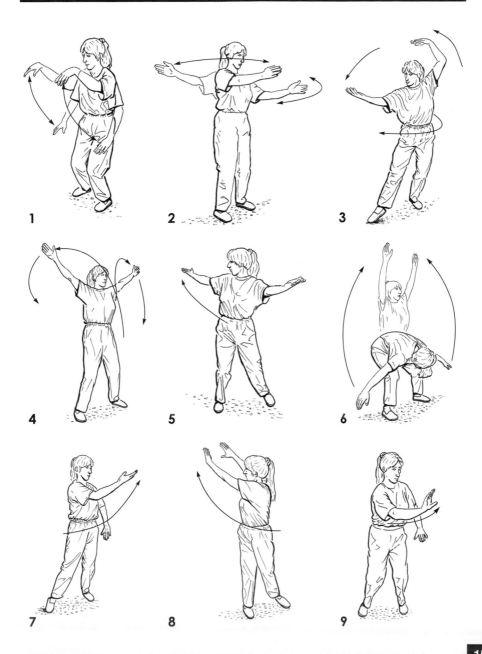

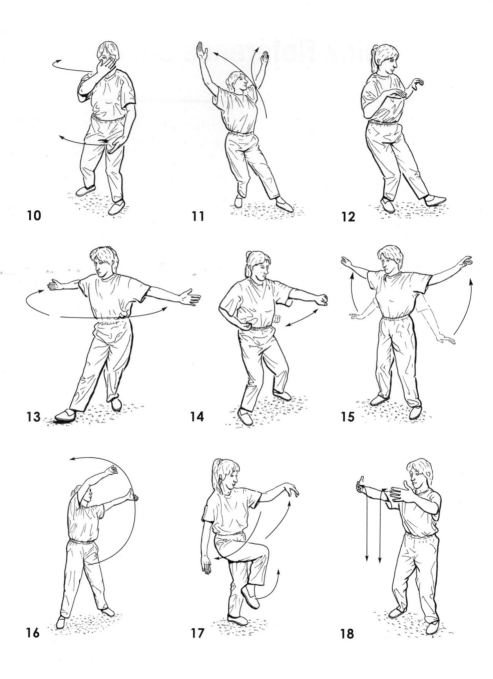